Eat Smart
and
Stay Slim

Eat Smart and Stay Slim

The GI Diet

Liesbet Delport RD (SA)
Gabi Steenkamp RD (SA)

Tafelberg

First published in 2003 by
Tafelberg Publishers Ltd
28 Wale Street, Cape Town 8000
Registration nr.: 51/02378/06

10 9 8 7 6 5 4 3

Publisher Anita Pyke
Editor Pat Barton
Index Lizé Lübbe
Illustration (page 24) Izak Vollgraaf
Design and Typesetting Alinea Studio, Cape Town

Printed and bound by Paarl Print,
Oosterland Str., Paarl, South Africa

ISBN 0 624041891

This book is dedicated to all those who've been on so many diets that they've given up hope of ever achieving permanent weight loss. We believe this will be the last book you'll ever have to read about weight loss and achieving your ideal body mass.

Acknowledgements

We'd like to thank both our secretaries for all the hours they spent putting the manuscript into the correct format.

Rhynette Hugo RD (SA), Jeske Wellman RD (SA) and Sorine Swanepoel RD (SA) deserve a huge thank you for their part in translating various parts of the manuscript.

We would also like to express our gratitude to our husbands and children; without your sacrifices and support, this book would never have been completed.

To Anita Pyke, our publisher, thank you for your patience and your faith in us.

We would like to acknowledge Diane Hampton, author of *The Diet Alternative*, who was our inspiration when we wrote the first section of this book.

We humbly acknowledge the hand of the Lord in the writing of this book.

Contents

Section 2
Low-GI, lower-fat eating
What should you eat?

Section 3
Activity

Chapter 9: Start exercising

Section 4
Recipes

Section 5
GI logos and lists

Foreword

I'm a new person!

Two years ago, Judy van Bergen (one of the editorial staff at *Huisgenoot*) changed her eating pattern to include mainly low-GI foods. She bought our recipe book, *Eating for Sustained Energy*, and made some small, but important, changes in her food choices. Within six months she had lost all her excess weight. This is her story:

Exactly two years ago I decided, "So far, and no further!" I was already overweight before I became pregnant with my son, and after his birth I was even heavier. Then the article on the Glycemic Index and a new way of eating, published in *Huisgenoot* (11 January 2001), caught my eye. The article was about the most popular diet in the country, devised by Liesbet Delport (a registered dietician), who advocated a balanced, low-GI, lower-fat diet, and it was an inspiration.

I've always been interested in diets, but had never had very successful results. With this diet, I realised, all I had to change was my eating pattern. I didn't really believe the weight would just melt away, as the article promised. But choosing to eat foods that kept me full for longer made sense, and it worked! It was so easy.

A lot of things suddenly became clear. I realised that it was the fat on the meat and the cheese on my bread that were making me fat; that a little sugar on my cereal was quite acceptable; and that I had the freedom to eat jam on my bread every now and then. It was wonderful! The recipe book was next to the stove every evening when I prepared dinner. The kilograms simply melted away; every week I lost about half a kilogram and the centimetres also disappeared. Within six months I had lost 8 kg. The compliments came streaming in … I was a new person!

Never before had it been so easy to lose weight. For the first time it didn't cost a fortune, and I didn't once find the diet difficult to follow. I was so impressed that I began chatting to readers in other towns. Their efforts were so successful that some of them even started their own clubs.

I'm now at the end of my first year. Eating for sustained energy has become a way of life, and I recommend this wonderful way of eating to everyone who wants to live healthily and would like the bonus of losing weight.

Judy van Bergen, *Huisgenoot*

Introduction

Do you often dream of getting slim and staying that way, without having to be on a diet forever? Wouldn't it be wonderful if food and weight no longer ruled your life, but became a normal part of it? Do you sometimes wish you could eat what you like, when you like, and as much as you like?

If you do, this book is for you!

Unfortunately, there's no magic formula for losing weight; we can also not give you licence to over-indulge. But we do believe it is possible to lose weight and maintain the weight loss. All you have to do is follow the principles outlined in this book; listen to your body and not eat for emotional reasons; adapt your lifestyle to eating a lower-fat diet, according to the Glycemic Index; and exercise regularly.

Overweight and obesity have become an enormous problem in today's world. More than 56% of South African women and 29% of South African men (of all race groups) are overweight, i.e. they weigh up to 10% more than their ideal body mass. Furthermore,

28% of South African women and 10% of South African men, of all race groups, are obese, i.e. they have a Body Mass Index (BMI) greater than 30.

The Body Mass Index (BMI) is calculated as follows:

$$\frac{\text{Body mass in kilograms (kg)}}{\text{Height (m) x Height (m)}}$$

So, for example, a woman who is 1,64 metres (164 cm) tall and weighs 70 kg, is overweight. For her height, she should weigh 55 kg and she is thus 15 kg (or 27%) heavier than her ideal weight. If the same woman weighed 82 kg, she would be classified as obese, because her BMI is greater than 30.

$$\frac{82}{1,64 \times 1,64} \longrightarrow 30$$

The multi-million-dollar slimming business doesn't seem to be helping those who are overweight; in fact, the number of overweight people worldwide increases every day. Overweight and obesity are now regarded as diseases, as they are associated with health problems such as high cholesterol levels, high blood pressure, diabetes, hyper-insulinaemia and insulin resistance, arthritis and gout, to mention just a few.

If diets, slimming programmes and diet products worked, there would surely not be so many overweight people in the world. So what's the problem? Why do people become overweight; why are there so many overweight people; why don't all these diets work; and why do people battle to keep off the weight they've lost? Research done by the Medical Research Council (MRC) and others has found that being overweight is a complex interaction between diet, environment and genetic factors. It may also be linked to cultural perceptions of body image, as well as access to food and exercise.

One of the reasons overweight people battle to lose weight and keep it off is that diet, on its own, cannot be the entire solution. So if you want to lose weight and maintain the weight loss, you will have to address these three equally important aspects:

14

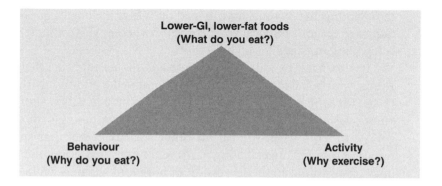

Lower-GI, lower-fat foods
(What do you eat?)

Behaviour
(Why do you eat?)

Activity
(Why exercise?)

◆ You will have to change your food choices, *permanently*. Fat, unfortunately, makes fat, which is why it's impossible to lose weight on a high-fat diet, unless you eat very little. In this book, we've included a fat questionnaire (page 95) for you to fill in, so you can find out what the fat content of your daily diet is. This is followed by many tips for reducing the quantity of fat in your diet, without sacrificing volume or taste.

◆ The GI (or Glycemic Index) measures, on a scale from 1 – 100, how much a carbohydrate-containing food (starches, dairy products, legumes, vegetables, fruit and sweets) will affect blood glucose levels. This brings us to the low-GI, lower-fat diet.

Low-GI foods (1 – 55 GI) release their glucose slowly and steadily into the bloodstream. It's easier to lose weight if you eat such foods because they keep you full for longer (about three hours). Eating low-GI foods also helps combat hyperinsulinaemia and insulin resistance, which are present in most overweight people. Both hyperinsulinaemia and insulin resistance make weight loss very difficult, because insulin stores fat. Foods with an intermediate GI (56 – 69 GI) release glucose into the blood stream a little faster (keeping you full for about two hours), while foods with a high GI release glucose into the bloodstream fairly quickly and offer satiety for a maximum of one hour. High-GI foods (above 70) result in sustained high blood glucose levels in diabetics, and can elicit a reactive hypoglycaemic response in healthy people, but especially in those who suffer from hypoglycaemia/low blood glucose. High-GI foods are recommended after exercise, however. To find out more about this and everything you need to know about the Glycemic Index, you'll have to read on! We've included a questionnaire (page 73) to help you determine whether you eat mostly low-, intermediate- or high-GI foods.

◆ You'll also have to look at your *reasons* for eating; in other words, your behaviour. Again, we have compiled a questionnaire (page 19) which will help you determine whether you eat for emotional reasons or in response to true hunger. Eating habits get out of hand when you eat for other reasons, rather than in response to true hunger. Eating in response to feeling hurt, loneliness, frustration, anger, depression or boredom will only aggravate an overweight problem. And trying to eat cucumber slices when you experience these emotions won't solve your problem, as you're still eating. As soon as you're no longer "on diet", you'll probably eat chocolates, chips and other high-fat, high-kilojoule foods again, which means you will regain any weight you may have lost. What you have to learn to do is to take the right "medicine" for your emotional problem (for example, calling a friend when you're feeling hurt) instead of using food to try to solve it. If you persevere, you will eventually get out of the habit of eating to compensate for emotional distress, and only eat when you are truly hungry, as all slim people do. Then you'll no longer tell yourself, "I'm not allowed to eat this or that", but rather, "I don't *want* to eat this or that because I'm not actually hungry"! Doing this will guarantee permanent weight loss.

◆ Last, but not least, you have to become more *active* (if you aren't already active enough). Most overweight people eat as though they've just run a marathon, when in reality they sit still most of the day, and this means they're consuming more than they need. Exercise increases your metabolic rate so you burn up more energy, and results in the release of endorphins, which make you feel better and help you not to overeat. To find out more about the advantages of exercising, see page 175. We've also included a questionnaire (page 169) to help you find out just how active you are.

Permanent weight loss *is* possible, and there are many living examples to prove the point. If you'd like to know more about the three important keys to permanent weight loss, read on. You won't regret it!

Behaviour

Why do you eat?

Chapter 1

Eating habits: who is in control?

Eating behaviour questionnaire

Do you eat in response to body needs, or for other reasons?

Read each question and choose the answer (from A to E) you agree with *most*:

A: don't agree at all
B: don't completely agree
C: sometimes agree, sometimes not
D: mostly agree
E: agree 100%

If you choose A, you agree *least* with the question; if you choose E, you agree *most*. Circle the number under the headings A to E that you've chosen as your answer. Add these numbers up after you've completed the questionnaire to get your total score, then check your results in "How did you score?"

		Agree with least				Agree with most
		A	B	C	D	E
1	I only eat when I am hungry	5	4	3	2	1
2	I never eat when I am bored	5	4	3	2	1
3	I often eat when I am depressed	1	2	3	4	5
4	When I am angry, I have to eat something	1	2	3	4	5
5	When I am lonely, I often eat chocolate	1	2	3	4	5
6	When I am tense, I cannot eat at all	5	4	3	2	1
7	I only eat to stay alive	5	4	3	2	1
8	I find it easy to fast	5	4	3	2	1
9	I only eat because I have to	5	4	3	2	1
10	I mostly eat when I am frustrated	1	2	3	4	5
11	Eating is one of the nicest things in life for me	1	2	3	4	5
12	I wish I could eat as much as I wanted to, without gaining weight	1	2	3	4	5
13	When I cannot sleep at night, I eat	1	2	3	4	5
14	I cannot read without something to eat	1	2	3	4	5
15	When watching TV at night, I have to eat	1	2	3	4	5
16	It is impossible for me not to eat, when other people around me are eating	1	2	3	4	5
17	I always clean my plate	1	2	3	4	5
18	I often forget to eat	5	4	3	2	1
19	I often buy myself something nice to eat, when driving past a café or bakery	1	2	3	4	5
20	When it is raining, I have to snack constantly	1	2	3	4	5

How did you score?

0 – 55: You probably don't have an eating problem and are definitely not a compulsive eater. You usually eat when you're hungry, and stop eating when you've had enough. Food doesn't bother you. You're in control of your eating habits and of food. Food doesn't control your life; it's only one of your interests. Your body weight is probably within the correct range for your height, unless you suffer from one or other medical condition such as hyperinsulinemia and insulin resistance or an underactive thyroid or are on medication that affects your weight e.g. hormone replacement therapy (HRT), cortisone or the like.

56 – 69: Beware! You're not a compulsive eater yet, but could easily become one because you love food and eating. You're probably slightly overweight, unless you're blessed with a very good metabolism. You don't eat only when you're hungry, but often for emotional reasons, or out of habit. See page 36 to find out how to get rid of compulsive behaviour.

70+: You're probably a compulsive eater and need help. Read the whole of Section 1 on behaviour and complete all the questionnaires. These guidelines will help you change your compulsive behaviour and take control of food and eating, rather than having it control your life.

Chapter 2

The problem: you are not in control

Hunger and satiety

There's a specific time and place for most things in life. For example, we use the bathroom to wash and relieve ourselves, and generally don't use it for any other purpose. We wouldn't go to the bathroom just because we felt like it, or because we were experiencing some negative emotion. But many people eat inappropriately to compensate for anger, depression, boredom, etc. Meals should be eaten at table, when you are hungry, using a plate and cutlery, and enjoyed until you are satisfied. If you stick to this guideline, you'll eliminate unnecessary eating and lose weight too!

 Do you only eat when you are hungry?

How your body works

The human body is a perfect biological system, and has all the most effective safety mechanisms and control systems in place. If you ignore the way your body is supposed to function and do things that may harm it – eating too much or too little, for instance – problems may arise. Overweight and obesity are results of bad habits, and will influence your body's ability to function optimally.

The human body is designed in such a way that it will digest and absorb food eaten at different rates. If you eat the right type of food, in the correct quantities, you'll have a constant flow of energy for up to five hours. If you eat the way that most modern people do, you won't have this sustained source of energy. The result is that you'll run out of energy (fuel) at the most inconvenient times of the day.

Your body needs fuel every 5 – 6 hours, and that's why, in most countries, it is the custom to eat three meals a day. If you don't eat the right types of food, in the correct quantities, you'll get hungry and need to eat between meals. This means you're taking in extra energy (fuel), which may result in weight gain, and this is the reason we recommend three meals a day, with *small* snacks in between, only if necessary (see page 165 for examples of snacks).

Research has shown that the sensation of hunger is preceded by a drop in blood sugar levels. Hunger is a sign that blood glucose levels have dropped and that glucose may no longer be immediately available. As a result, you will feel the need to "refuel" (eat) to ensure a source of fuel for the body.

What about the snacking theory, you may ask?

A lot of people cannot eat a full meal at one sitting, because they're satisfied too soon. They might want to eat smaller meals every 2 – 3 hours. This means they'll eat bigger snacks than someone who eats three larger meals a day. If you watch these "snackers" closely, you'll see most of them have a normal body weight. This is because they're very sensitive to the signs of hunger and satiety, and eat only as much as their body needs with every "mini-meal".

The problem with most overweight people is that they use the snacking theory as an excuse to eat all the time. The difference between these people and snackers who are a normal weight, is that they have no idea when they're really hungry and eat mainly because they feel like eating, purely from habit. They usually also make poor food choices, eating high-fat, high-GI foods that will only aggravate their problem.

Stop eating when you are satisfied

Hunger and satiety centre

Hunger and satiety are primitive, inborn instincts for which there are control centres in the hypothalamus of humans and animals (see figure below). There's a "feeding centre" to one side of the hypothalamus and a "satiety centre" in the centre. When the "feeding centre" of animals used for research was destroyed, it led to anorexia (loss of appetite), and lesions to the "satiety centre" resulted in a dramatic increase in hunger. This shows that the centres are programmed to send signals that will let us know when we're hungry (and need energy/fuel) and when we're satisfied (and have to stop eating). This works very well when we're babies; a baby will cry when it's hungry, thirsty, tired, wet, etc. The mother has to determine what the problem is as soon as possible and solve it. If the baby is wet and is fed, he or she will still be uncomfortable and will continue crying because the initial problem has not been solved. If a baby is hungry or thirsty and gets fed, the correct solution has been provided and the baby will stop crying and be content.

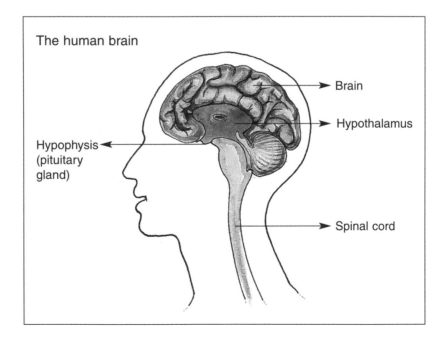

The human brain

Brain

Hypothalamus

Hypophysis (pituitary gland)

Spinal cord

Incorrect programming

Over time, some people get into the habit of eating and drinking when they're not really hungry or thirsty, and their body's satiety and hunger control is disturbed. Unfortunately, many of us get this incorrect programming from our parents, and we pass it on to our children in turn. When a child is upset, we normally comfort him or her with a biscuit or sweet, instead of a hug or a "kiss-it-better". When a child falls and hurts itself, a plaster and a little comforting are all that should be required. Yet many mothers insist on giving the child something to eat as well. Disappointed and hurt teenagers are often comforted if we take them out for a meal, when we should rather let them pour their heart out, or allow them to cry and then comfort them.

You can even programme yourself incorrectly. Every time you eat when you're not really hungry, you add to the problem. The more often you eat without being hungry, the more you suppress your hunger and satiety centre, until it can no longer function properly.

One of our patients had a similar problem. He was a train driver who hated using the public toilets on the train. Every time he had an urge to use the bathroom, he would suppress it until it disappeared. Since he worked on the train all day for many years, his body stopped sending him the signal that he needed to use the bathroom, and the end result was constipation. His body will probably only start functioning properly again once he stops working and knows he can use a clean bathroom at any time of the day. In the same way, you can "unlearn" listening to your body's satiety signals, if you eat all day long.

Genetic factors: the good news and the bad news

Most overweight people who have overweight parents and grandparents think they have a genetic predisposition to obesity. Genetics and your medical history *do* play a role in how much you weigh, but the relationship is not that simple.

Even though overweight is inclined to run in families, it may simply be the result of poor eating habits learnt in that family. According to Dr Bridget Farham, there's no reason why you should remain overweight (like the rest of your family), if you're prepared to take control of your lifestyle. Although there are people who suffer from metabolic abnormalities, they're in the minority and can usually be helped with special medications, such as those that correct abnormal thyroid function.

The bad news, then, is that no one will get slim and stay slim unless they learn to listen to their body's signals of hunger and satiety. The good news is that you can relearn listening to your body's signals that you're full, and it's time to stop eating. Don't blame your parents for programming you incorrectly. Start today by asking yourself this question every time you want to eat something: "Am I really hungry, or am I eating because I have another problem?" You'll be surprised at how positive the results are!

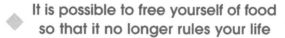

It is possible to free yourself of food so that it no longer rules your life

Where does compulsive eating come from?

We believe that the natural response to eat when we are hungry and to stop eating when we are full gets distorted when we eat for emotional and other reasons. This is the start of compulsive eating and comprises one "leg" on which it stands. Most of the statements listed below will sound familiar to you, if you are a compulsive eater.

Emotional reasons for eating:
- I feel lonely today, so I'll reward myself with a packet of biscuits.
- The staff have already made me angry, even though it's still early, so I deserve a packet of biltong or dried wors.
- I've had such a stressful day, I need a few beers to relax tonight.
- I can't master this accounting course and it's really frustrating. I'm sure I'll feel better once I've eaten a packet of chips with dipping sauce and had a large cooldrink.

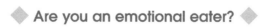

Are you an emotional eater?

Physical reasons for eating:
- I worked really hard this morning, so I need a chocolate to replenish all the energy I've used up.

◆ I'll have to study all night and I'm already tired. I deserve a midnight snack.
◆ Today I have to drive all day and I know I'll get very sleepy, so I need to eat to stay awake.

Circumstantial or social reasons that may lead to overeating:
◆ I'm at a tea party where everyone's eating cake and other delicacies. I can't *not* eat, so I'll just have to join in.
◆ I've already eaten supper because I didn't know there'd be food at this function. But it all looks so delicious that I'll have to try some.
◆ It's normal to eat more than usual at the weekend.
◆ When I'm on holiday, I don't want to be restricted in any way, least of all with my food.
◆ When we have visitors, I don't have time to think about what I eat.
◆ When I'm visiting other people, it's impossible to eat according to my body's needs.
◆ This week we'll be eating out three times, so I'll definitely pick up weight.
◆ Friday nights are my nights out with my friends at the pub. I can't refuse them.
◆ While I'm studying for exams, I concentrate better if I constantly nibble something.
◆ I'm so bored. I'm sure a slab of chocolate will make me feel better.

These are just a few examples. Try to identify the circumstances, emotions and social occasions that make you overeat for the wrong reasons and write them down in the table below. We've filled in one example for you.

Reason for eating or drinking	Emotion, physical reason or circumstance
I'm feeling sorry for myself because my friend just left me.	Self-pity

The habit of eating

The tendency to eat for the wrong reasons is the main cause of compulsive eating. The more often you do it, the more firmly the habit takes hold, until you reach the point where you no longer listen to your body and hardly ever eat because you're really hungry. In fact, you find it difficult to differentiate between real hunger and whether you just feel like eating as a result of your appetite, boredom, etc. You're no longer in control of what you eat; in fact, the opposite is true: food and eating have taken control of your life. You've now developed the *habit* of eating, and this forms the other "leg" on which compulsive eating rests (remember, the first "leg" is eating for the wrong reasons). Let us explain.

Examples of habitual eating:
◆ Eating every time you walk past the fridge or the kitchen. Just as it would be ridiculous to go to the toilet every time you walk past

the bathroom, so should it seem silly to eat every time you walk past the fridge or the kitchen (once you've broken the habit of compulsive eating, of course).

◆ When you open a packet of biscuits, chips or a slab of chocolate, you have to continue eating until it's all gone.

◆ When others around you are eating, you have to join in.

◆ When you open a packet of chips, you can't put it down until it's finished.

◆ When you go out drinking with friends, you end up having at least five beers without even realising it.

◆ You have to keep tasting the food while you're cooking.

◆ You always end up eating your baby's leftovers.

◆ When baking rusks, you have to gather up and eat all the crumbs and bits that break off.

◆ When asked by your host if you'd like another helping, you always have more, even though you've had enough.

◆ You eat three meals a day with snacks in between, not because you're hungry, but because you always do so.

◆ The smell of freshly baked bread always lures you into the bakery to buy something, and eat it, even though you're not hungry.

We think you'll agree that, in order to free yourself from habitual eating and eating for the wrong reasons, you'll have to take some drastic steps. We're convinced you *can* break free from being controlled by food and eating, but in order to do so, you'll have to ditch habitual eating. Read on to find out how.

The list above gives only a few examples. In the table below write down some of your own "habitual eating" habits – times when you end up eating, not because you're hungry, but because it's a bad habit.

Again, we've given you one example.

Behaviour: why do you eat?

It's lunchtime and time to eat (even though I had three pieces of cake at teatime because it was a colleague's birthday, and I cannot possibly be hungry)

Chapter 3

The solution: shifting the "C" from compulsive eating to controlled eating

It's very important to identify those compulsive eating patterns that keep you from losing weight. As soon as you've identified them (and you'll uncover more every day), you need to find alternative behaviour patterns to substitute for your poor habits and help you overcome them. Remember that these new habits or activities must be pleasurable experiences, so you'll continue with them for the rest of your life.

How to get out of the habit of eating

Perhaps you're thinking: "I'm already in the habit of eating all the time, mainly for the wrong reasons, but how do I free myself of the control food and eating have over me? How do I make food just one of the important issues in my life, not the overriding one?"

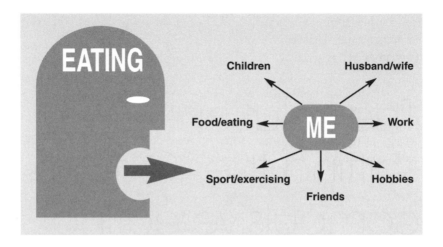

Eat only three meals a day

Our bodies are programmed to need re-fuelling every 5 – 6 hours. For this reason we recommend that you try to stick to eating only three meals a day. Try to eat every meal sitting down at table, using crockery and cutlery. After breakfast, say to yourself that you've finished eating, you're no longer hungry and the next meal will be lunch. Eating is no longer on the agenda for the morning. Now consult your "to do" list and get cracking. Drinking between meals is not a problem as long as you stick to drinks low in kilojoules (calories). Water, artificially sweetened cooldrinks, tea or coffee with skimmed milk or low-fat milk – preferably without sugar or sweetened with sweetener – are all suitable. Then apply the same principles after lunch and dinner.

This new habit of "fasting" between meals will help you get out of the habit of eating, as your jaws are no longer working constantly for 3 – 5 hours! Remember that the habit of eating is one of the "legs" on which compulsive eating stands. By merely cutting out all the in-between eating, you should already begin to lose weight. You'll also begin to be able to distinguish between true hunger and mere appetite.

Should you really get hungry after 3 – 4 hours (not after 1 hour, unless you've eaten incorrectly), you could eat a piece of fruit as a snack. You'll see, in the menu section (page 156), that we've differentiated between "snack snacks" and "meal snacks". If you've eaten a "snack snack" between meals, you can still eat your three meals for that day. If you chose to eat a "meal snack", however, you'll have to compensate for this larger snack at the next meal (see page 164).

At first, you'll think you're hungry, but if you persevere you'll find that you cope quite adequately with this regimen. Two main meals with one "meal snack" (and perhaps two or three "snack snacks") will be more than enough for a day. As you progress, you will no longer feel that "this is all I'm allowed to eat", but rather that "this is all I *can* eat, as I am actually full"!

Change bad eating habits gradually

Rome wasn't built in a day, and you won't get slim overnight. It takes time to break the bad habits acquired over many years in order to lose weight, but the results should be permanent.

Use the table below to write down the circumstances, situations or activities that you link with eating, as well as the new habits you will try to substitute for the bad eating habits.

We've filled in one example to help you on your way.

Circumstances, situations or activities that lead to eating	Changes that will eventually help you not to link these situations with eating
While reading a book, I have to have coffee and chocolate	I will try to drink water only for the first hour

A practical activity to help you break bad (eating) habits:

The purpose of this activity is to help you achieve, and maintain, healthy eating habits. The steps outlined below will guide you in: identifying areas of improvement; setting a goal; and developing a plan of action.

1. Identifying areas for improvement. We encourage you to use information from your most recent food record or self-monitoring and/or past experience to identify areas for dietary improvement. List the three areas that are most important to you from a personal perspective.

1. _____

2. _____

3. _____

2. Setting a goal. Select an area for dietary modification from the list above. Your goal must be specific, measurable and realistic. Answer all questions that apply to the area you've selected for modification.
Area to modify:
What will you do differently so that you know (or someone else observing you knows) that you're making progress toward your goal? Be specific.

Specify time period (e.g. week, month, vacation, etc.):

_____

Specify how often (e.g. daily, once a week, etc.):

_____

Specify how much (e.g. 125 ml [$^1/_2$ C], 30 g, etc.):

_____

Specify where (e.g. at home, at work, in a restaurant, at a function, etc.):

_____

Specify with whom (e.g. husband, children, grandchildren, friends, etc.):

_____

3. Developing a plan of action. List the three challenges you're most likely to encounter in striving for your dietary goal.

Challenge 1

_____

Challenge 2

_____

Challenge 3

_____

What will you do to manage your challenges, in order, to prevent their affecting your ability to attain your goal?

To manage challenge 1, I will

_____

To manage challenge 2, I will

_____

To manage challenge 3, I will

_____

How confident are you, on a scale of 0 – 100%, that you can achieve this goal?

(0%) (10%) (20%) (30%) (40%) (50%)

(60%) (70%) (80%) (90%) (100%)

If you're not at least 75% confident, modify your goal to increase the likelihood that you will be successful.

I will begin working on the following goal: _____

_____

on (date) _____. I will monitor myself using an eating diary to evaluate my success in reaching this goal. I will bring the diary with me to my next appointment and discuss successes/ challenges with my dietician.

Signature: _____

Date: _____

Taken from: _Facilitating Dietary Change: The Patient-centered Counseling Model_, by M.C. Rosal, PhD; C.B. Ebbeling, PhD; I.S. Ockene, MD and J.R. Hebert, Dsc

Stop eating for the wrong reasons

Whenever you find yourself wanting to eat and it isn't time to eat and you're not hungry, *do something*.

When you wake up in the morning, try asking yourself what you will do today, not what you'll eat today. Although one does have to plan meals for the day, this shouldn't be your only concern. Then, when you want to eat, first refer to your list of things to do and get on with one of them. The more you do things when you want to eat even though you're not hungry, the more control you'll gain over food and eating. In this way you will gradually "paralyse" this second "leg" – eating for the wrong reasons – on which compulsive eating stands, until it eventually gives way.

It won't help to eat lettuce and cucumber when you're bored, because you will still be eating for the wrong reason. If you're not really hungry and you feel the urge to eat, you need to do something else to free yourself from the bonds of food and eating. When you get up in the morning, rather have a shower or bath first and wait until you're at least a little hungry before you have breakfast. It *is* important to eat regular meals, but it will be very difficult to know when you've had enough to eat if you weren't hungry in the first place. The more you put other activities first, the weaker the hold food has on you will become. With time, you'll find you cannot eat if you aren't hungry.

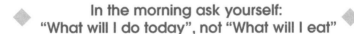

**In the morning ask yourself:
"What will I do today", not "What will I eat"**

It requires 30 consecutive efforts of changed behaviour to see any progress.

According to psychologists, one has to repeat a new activity 30 times to form a new habit. Let's look at an example. Imagine that you have a bad habit – say, biting your nails – and you wish to get rid of it. If you started knitting every time you wanted to bite your nails, you'd find that, after 30 times of substituting the new behaviour, you would automatically knit when you wanted to bite your nails. Should you bite your nails again after the fifth time or so that you've substituted the new behaviour, however, you'd have to start all over again, and continue until you started knitting for 30 consecutive times when you felt the urge to bite your nails. Then you will have formed a new habit. In the same way, the more you train yourself do to something else whenever you want to eat, and you do this for 30 consecutive times, the easier it will be to get rid of the habit of eating for the wrong reasons.

What are the things you would still *like* to do (things you enjoy doing)? Fill them in below (we've given you an example).

I'd like to stick all my photos in an album

Fill in below all the things that you still *have* to do (again, we've provided an example)

I have to make new curtains for my kitchen

Whenever you're in a situation that increases your chances of overeating, move to a situation where you forget about food.

Fill in the table below, listing in the left-hand column all the circumstances, situations and activities that encourage you to eat. In the right-hand column list those activities, situations or circumstances that help you to forget about food. Whenever you find yourself in a situation listed in the left-hand column (one that encourages you to eat), try to change it to one in the right-hand column (something that helps you forget about food). See page 49 for creative and other activities that may help you to forget about food.

An example has been filled in for you.

Circumstances/situations/ activities that tempt me to eat	Circumstances/situations/activities that help me forget about food
When I do the grocery shopping	When I'm sewing a new dress

Shift your focus

Remember: Your main aim is to ensure that food and eating no longer control your life, and that food takes its rightful place in your life as one of a number of other interests. We have already discussed the first few important points to help you achieve this goal, and now we come to another.

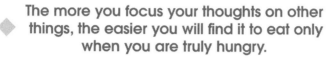

The more you focus your thoughts on other things, the easier you will find it to eat only when you are truly hungry.

Slimming diets: the traditional focus

The main aim of slimming diets is to lose weight. Most slimmers weigh themselves nearly every day, and many weigh themselves two or three times a day. This serves no purpose, except to focus attention on the scale, your weight and ultimately on food and eating – which is precisely what you *don't* want. On many slimming diets, the dieter focuses so much on which foods must be eaten, which are forbidden, the weighing of food, etc. that the tendency to focus on food increases.

We're sure you'll agree that the life of most slimmers revolves around their weight and the scale, as well as food and eating. Does the following situation sound familiar? When you get up on Monday morning you weigh 2 kg more than you did before the weekend. You decide to "go on diet" and by Friday you've lost only 1 kg. You are now so annoyed and frustrated that you give up and start overeating again. Or you see that you have lost 3 kg by Friday, so you reward yourself with the freedom to eat as much as you like over the weekend. You have to agree that this mindset will never help anyone to stay slim.

Re-focus

If you want food and eating to lose their control over you, you cannot let the scale and your weight continue to be your central focus. To learn to listen to your body's signals telling you when you're full or when you're hungry, you will have to lose your obsession with food, eating, your weight and the scale.

The scale merely shows you your body weight, which is only a symptom of your actual problem – that food and eating control your life. In order to shift the "C" from compulsive to controlled eating, you have to change your focus. The less control food and eating have over you, the less you will weigh on the scale; it's inevitable! Begin working towards weighing yourself once a week only, listening to your body, and only eating when you are truly hungry. Try also to assess your body weight by the way your clothes fit, rather than by weighing yourself frequently.

To achieve your new goals, try to focus on the following.

◆ Make a decision *now* that you won't think about food as soon as you wake up, but rather focus on something else. Waiting until you're actually hungry before eating breakfast also helps to shift your focus from food.

◆ Make a conscious decision to focus your thoughts on other activities, such as your current hobby project, planning your garden for the next season, or rearranging a room. For more tips, see page 49.

◆ Whenever you catch yourself thinking or fantasising about food, decide *immediately* to think of something else. The human brain has difficulty remembering anything negative. So don't tell yourself, "I mustn't eat any cake" because you'll still be thinking about cake. If you're then confronted with the reality of eating cake, you won't be able to resist. Have you ever wondered why a young girl in the throes of love loses weight easily? Because she's thinking of her loved one constantly and completely forgets to eat.

The more you train your thoughts to focus on other things the more often you'll forget about eating and, in time, begin eating only in response to true hunger and stop eating when you're full. And these behaviours are what will help you rid yourself of the control that food and eating have over you.

"Reprogramme" your brain

When it comes to food, most of us have been incorrectly programmed from childhood. Let's look at a few examples.

◆ You stub your toe and your mother gives you a biscuit to comfort you.

◆ You missed out at a school prize-giving, and are rewarded with a chocolate instead.

◆ Your friend hits you and your father buys you a cooldrink or ice cream.

What happens is that you now get the idea that emotional problems should be "medicated" with "comfort" foods. It doesn't have to stay this way; it *is* possible to reprogramme yourself, if you really want to.

A few positive thoughts are listed below. Try to read some or all of them every day or – even better – to say them out loud. This will help to reprogramme your brain so that when you feel hurt and want the comfort of a packet of biscuits, for instance, you remember that you should only eat when you're hungry and not in response to the hurt you're feeling. It may sound rather odd, but hearing yourself saying these thoughts out loud helps to reprogramme your brain and convince you of the truth of what you're saying.

1. I don't live to eat; I eat to stay alive.
2. My life doesn't revolve around eating. Eating is something I do two or three times a day, when I'm hungry and until I'm full.
3. Eating is not the only pleasure in my life. It's one of my interests and is currently taking its rightful place in my life.
4. I don't get fulfilment from food. I get fulfilment from my hobbies (reading, sewing, woodwork, etc.), my sport (running, swimming, walking, aerobics, etc.) and from doing things for other people, or spending time with them (chatting with a friend, spending time with my child, etc.). These things feed my soul.
5. I don't have to eat more just because it's the weekend or we're on holiday. I eat only when I am hungry and only until I am full.
6. I mustn't give up working on my eating habits just because I overdid it. I forgive myself and from this moment on, I will try again. I do *not* have to wait until tomorrow or Monday.
7. I have the rest of my life to eat every day. I don't have to eat it all today.
8. I'm not on a diet; I'm learning to eat according to my body's needs, not according to whim.

Setting goals to change eating habits

There are four steps to successful goal setting.

Step 1: Acknowledge the need to change

It's very important that before you try to lose weight, you realise that you need to lose weight, or that there is a problem with your eating habits and that they need to be changed. This is especially true if you scored more than 55 points (and especially if you scored more than 70 points) when you filled in the questionnaire at the beginning of this section (page 20). Use the tables below to determine whether your Body Mass Index (BMI) falls within the healthy range, whether your waist/hip ratio is normal and whether your body fat percentage is normal for your age. If your BMI is above 30 and your waist/hip ratio and body fat percentage are above the normal ranges, you do need to lose weight.

Body Mass Index (BMI) =	$\dfrac{\text{Mass in kilograms (kg)}}{\text{Height (m) x Height (m)}}$

(See also the example in the Introduction, page 14)

Ideal BMI values:	
Gender	**Ideal BMI**
Women	19 – 24
Men	20 – 25

If your BMI is below the recommended values, you're underweight. If it's above 25, you're classed as overweight, but if it's over 30, you're *very* overweight and would be classed as obese.

The waist/hip ratio in women should be 0,8. For example, a woman who has a waist measurement of 64 cm should have a hip measurement of 80 cm. In contrast, men should have a waist/hip ratio of 1,0. So a man with a waist measurement of 65 cm should have a hip measurement of 65 cm. Men with a waist/hip ratio of more than 1,0 are far more likely to suffer from cardiovascular diseases than those with a ratio of 1,0 or less.

There are two methods of determining **body fat percentage:** using a special scale or electrodes, and using calipers. Calipers measure the amount of fat under the skin. A biokineticist can determine the percentage of body fat accurately, using the calipers and a special formula. The body fat percentage should be as follows.

Ideal fat percentage for women (using calipers)			
Age	Active sportswomen	Normal	Inactive women
16 – 29	15 – 19%	21%	23 – 28%
30 – 39	16 – 21%	23%	25 – 30%
40+	18 – 23%	25%	27 – 32%

Ideal fat percentage for men (using calipers)			
Age	Active sportsmen	Normal	Inactive men
16 – 29	7 – 13%	15%	17 – 23%
30 – 39	9 – 15%	17%	19 – 25%
40+	10 – 17%	19%	21 – 28%

Special scales and electrodes measure the fat under your skin as well as the fat around your organs. Both personal trainers and dieticians can do this measurement for you. The values should be as follows.

Ideal fat percentages, using special electrodes or scales	
Gender	Ideal fat percentage
Women	21 – 34
Men	8 – 22

It's very important that body fat be measured at the same time of day, and preferably on the same day of the week and time of day. The person being measured should be well hydrated. For an accurate measurement, it's better to have body fat measured by a professional, and not do it yourself.

Section 2 of this book contains two questionnaires that will help you find out how you rate in terms of your fat intake and your average Glycemic Index (GI) rating. If your scores are higher than those recommended, it should also be an indication that you need to change your eating habits. Please also note the increased risks of high-fat, high-GI intakes and being overweight in terms of cardiovascular disease, diabetes, high blood pressure, etc .

Step 2: Formulate your goal

It's very important to formulate a goal that is specific, challenging and attainable, rather than one that's vague, boring and unattainable. Let's look at an example.

For argument's sake, let's imagine that you weigh 100 kg at the beginning of the year and your goal weight is 70 kg. It would be wiser to set your goal at losing 10 kg in the first quarter of the year, another 10 kg by the middle of the year, and the entire 30 kg by the end of the year, than to aim at losing the entire 30 kg within the first quarter. Losing 30 kg in three months is physically impossible, unless you are very hard on yourself and literally starve. In any case, this won't produce permanent results. If you lose between 500 g and 1 kg every week, you will reach your goal of getting slim and staying slim.

The advantage of setting more than one goal is that it focuses your attention and activities on your actions and habits, which means you can mobilise personal and social support systems. One is more inclined to put in effort once a goal has been set than when one has no goal at all.

Step 3: Monitor the activities that help you achieve your goals

Every plan must have checks and balances, and it's the same with setting goals. You, or preferably your dietician, should check regularly on your progress towards reaching your goal(s). If you're not reaching your goal(s) as planned, you may need to go back to Step 1 and consider whether you are indeed convinced of the need to change. You may also have to rethink your goal (Step 2) and perhaps simplify it, or adapt it to your eating behaviour so that it is possible to achieve. Read pages 50 – 52 on how to monitor your activities in order to reach your goal(s).

Step 4: Reward yourself for goals reached (not food-related rewards)

People who get rewards for achieving goals fare better than those who get no rewards. For this reason, we recommend that you keep daily records such as a food diary (i.e. write down what and how much you eat on every occasion) and pay weekly visits to a dietician who can monitor your progress and encourage you.

Changing eating habits

Step 1: Acknowledge the need to change
Step 2: Formulate your goal
Step 3: Monitor the activities that help you achieve your goals
Step 4: Reward yourself for goals reached

Learn to compensate

Compensating is something all naturally slim people do, yet very few people learn to compensate while they're trying to lose weight. This is especially true of fad diets, where rigid rules have to be adhered to.

If you observe naturally slim people, you'll notice that they often refuse food offered to them. If you ask them why they've refused an offer of food, they'll probably reply that they're not hungry, or they've just eaten lunch, or they ate too much at the last meal, or something else in the same vein. This is because they eat only in response to their hunger and satiety signals, and it's the reason they're always slim and never have to "go on diet". As we've said before, it *is* possible to relearn recognising these signals of hunger and satiety. One way to do so is to learn the art of compensating. Let's look at a few examples.

How to compensate when you've had breakfast at a hotel

Hotel breakfasts offer a huge, delicious variety of foods to choose from: breakfast cereals; fruit (fresh, dried, tinned, as well as fruit juices); dairy products such as milk, yoghurt and cheese; eggs and other protein dishes such as sausages, bacon and baked beans; vegetables such as tomatoes, onions and mushrooms; as well as baked delicacies such as breads, muffins, croissants and scones. Very few people would normally eat such a large and varied breakfast every day. In fact, if you go to Section 2 of this book, where we give you examples of the recommended quantities of food for each meal (page 117), you'll see that one hotel breakfast contains as much food as a normal breakfast and lunch put together – and that's only if you're eating circumspectly!

So, if you begin your hotel breakfast with cereal and milk or yoghurt, together with a few pieces of fruit, you've already eaten a full home breakfast. If you then have an egg dish and some other protein food, such as sausages, bacon or some baked beans, as well as tomatoes or mushrooms, then round off the meal with a few pastries with jam and cheese, you'll have to give up your lunch as well as the fruit you usually eat between meals.

This has nothing to do with dieting; the fact remains that you've eaten your breakfast, lunch and snacks in one sitting. If you're honest with yourself, and if you're in tune with your hunger and satiety centre, in a case such as this you'll find that you don't get hungry until late afternoon or suppertime. Of course, you can drink as many low-kilojoule drinks as you like throughout the day (water, artificially sweetened cooldrinks, tea and coffee [preferably decaffeinated] with low-fat or fat-free milk and sweetener or a touch of sugar). A normal supper should then be enough for the end of the day; you won't need a second helping as you've already eaten breakfast and lunch, only much earlier than usual.

If you find you get too hungry by late afternoon, perhaps it would be better for you to eat either the cereal, fruit and yoghurt/milk *or* the cooked eggs, sausage/bacon meal for your hotel breakfast. Doing this will allow you to have a small lunch, which will sustain you better throughout the afternoon. Whichever you choose, these tips should help you to maintain your weight if you're staying at a hotel while on holiday.

Having said this, it's still better to spread your food evenly throughout the day by eating breakfast, lunch and supper with small snacks in between, than to eat so much in one sitting. The reason is that your body is inclined to store fat more easily when the metabolic pathways are overloaded, as they would be if you ate too much in one go.

How to compensate when you've eaten a restaurant meal

When you know you're going to eat out later in the day, be it at a restaurant, or at a wedding or family gathering, you must try to eat less during the day (without letting your blood glucose levels drop too low). The reason for this is that eating-out portions of food are always much richer and bigger than foods prepared at home. You could try eating more low-GI vegetables at mealtimes during the day, especially at lunchtime, so that you don't arrive at the restaurant feeling hungry. A good idea is to eat a large low-GI salad before going out. Drinking more water and low-kilojoule drinks throughout the day will also ensure that you don't eat too much because you are, in fact, thirsty.

Ordering a ladies' portion and not feeling obliged to go through the whole menu also helps. Remember that each restaurant dish is often equivalent to a whole meal at home. If you then order a starter and a main course, you've eaten the equivalent of two meals at home (unless your starter was a low-fat vegetable dish such as French salad without dressing, or grilled mushrooms). So, in theory, you don't need breakfast the next morning. The same holds true if you eat a main meal and a dessert, since the dessert actually counts as your "breakfast". Of course, if you eat only half the main course to compensate for the dessert, you will need breakfast the next morning.

Ideally, you should stop eating when you're full and take the leftovers home in a "doggie bag". Eating only until you are full, not because the food's on your plate or there's so much available, will ensure that you don't pick up weight, even if eating out is on your agenda. You would also not have to give up your next meal, as you didn't overeat at the previous meal. But remember, in order to lose weight, you have to eat slightly less than you need. Remember, too, that all these principles we are teaching you are there to be followed for the rest of your life, even when you've become slim. We can't emphasise this enough!

How to compensate while on a cruise or package holiday

These must be the most difficult holidays to go on when you're trying to lose weight; even if you aren't, it's hard enough *not* to gain weight when you do not have control over what you are eating. Your best option is to try to avoid such holidays if you're trying to lose weight, but if this is not possible, try these tips.

◆ Follow our suggestions for the hotel breakfast in order to know what to do at breakfast time. If you want to eat lunch, have "half" a breakfast. If you've eaten a full breakfast, don't even go to the dining room at lunchtime, as your breakfast should keep you full until dinner. In such situations, one often eats in response to the look and smell of the food, not because one is hungry.

◆ If you're listening to your body, you should only get hungry towards dinnertime, when you can follow our suggestions for a restaurant meal. Should you wish to eat breakfast the next morning, you must eat only as much as you would eat at home, not several courses.

◆ Never partake of a midnight meal, unless you skipped dinner because you ate too much at breakfast or lunch that day. If you eat the midnight dinner, you definitely do *not* need breakfast the next morning.

The more you practise compensating, the easier it will become for you to listen to your body. It takes time to change eating habits, but the more you try, the quicker it becomes second nature to do so. Once you've learnt the art of listening to your body's hunger and satiety signals, nobody can take it away from you. It's a skill that goes with you wherever you are, unlike the scale, which you can't take everywhere with you.

The value of activity – creative and otherwise

The therapeutic benefits of creative activities are threefold: they keep your mind off food and eating, they give you a sense of achievement, and they keep your thoughts focused on interesting things.

Examples of creative activities

◆ Sewing/woodwork: One easily gets so engrossed in sewing or making a table, for example, that all thoughts of food and eating are banished.

◆ Gardening is a very therapeutic hobby for slimmers as it's not only creative but physical as well, especially when you plan and lay out a new garden. If you could go out and garden every time you thought about food or eating, you'd lose weight in no time at all.

◆ Playing a musical instrument: You're never too old to learn to play the musical instrument of your choice, even one that's not so well known, such as the clarinet. If you decide to learn to play a new musical instrument, it will keep you very busy because you'd like to progress as quickly as possible. If you practised playing your instrument every time you thought of food and were not really hungry, you'd lose weight and master the instrument pretty smartly. Learning to play an instrument also changes your focus.

◆ Woodcarving: Not many people practise this art, but why shouldn't you become one of them? There must be someone in your area who can give you lessons, or you could follow instructions from a book on woodcarving (from your local library) or from the Internet.

◆ Candlewicking, patchwork, crocheting, knitting and embroidery: These are all handicrafts that can give hours of pleasure. By following instructions from a book or from the Internet, or taking lessons, you could easily become an expert in any one of them. The best part is that you're distracted from thinking about food and eating, and will consequently learn to eat only in response to true hunger, i.e. three times a day, with two or three small snacks in between.

These are just a few examples of creative activities you could get involved in. Add your own on the next page, in particular those you've always wanted to try.

Find some other things you like doing and spoil yourself with these to help you get closer to your goal of only eating in response to true hunger. *Never* spoil yourself with food, and try not to combine any activity with eating.

Examples of non-food indulgences

◆ One of the most "delicious" things to do, once family and other obligations have been met, is to lie flat on your back and read a magazine. If you're lucky enough to have a hammock, you can make yourself very comfortable.

◆ There can be few pleasures in life quite as enjoyable as getting a novel (or whatever else you like to read) from the library before departing on holiday, and then spending the first day of your holiday engrossed in your book.

◆ Enjoying a nap on a Saturday or Sunday afternoon is a real treat. If you're on holiday, you could take a nap every day.

◆ And we haven't even mentioned the wonderful feeling of being spoilt when you lie in bed on a cold winter's day until you are thoroughly sick of being in bed.

◆ Chatting to a special friend is a great treat and it can be so fulfilling that you clean forget to eat.

These are just a few examples of spoiling yourself without involving food. Add some of your own below, especially those activities you find therapeutic and those you enjoy.

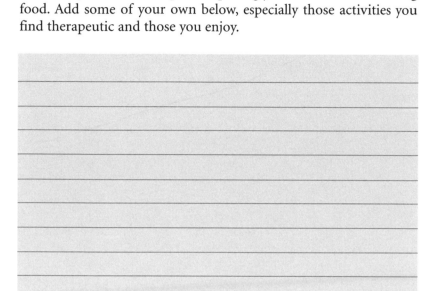

The best kind of activity to get involved in is physical activity; not only does it distract you from food and eating, but it also burns up energy.

Examples of physical activities
(See page 175 for the advantages of being active)

- Do a walking trail with your family, partner or friend(s) on a Saturday or Sunday.
- Train for a marathon, race or cycle tour and participate often; you'll find it very motivating and it will distract you from thoughts of food and eating.
- Join a sports club and play your sport, e.g. tennis, every weekend.
- When you feel frustrated, take a walk. Or walk regularly with a friend, your child, or your partner. If you don't get any other time to chat to them, this is the perfect time to enjoy a heart-to-heart. Good conversations are very possible while exercising!
- Learn to play golf and play at the weekend, if you feel the need to get out. But don't put back all the kilojoules you burnt off on the golf course at the 19th hole!

◆ Take dancing lessons. Dancing burns lots of energy without your realising it.

Again, these are just a few examples. Add a few more physical activities that you enjoy below.

Give up the food habit

Perhaps you've heard this said about an alcoholic: "As long as he sees the bottle as the solution to his problems or as his only friend, he won't be freed from alcoholism." This is very true; an alcoholic first has to acknowledge that alcohol is the problem, before he will seek help.

◆ **An alcoholic misuses alcohol;
a wine connoisseur appreciates it.** ◆

The same holds true for eating habits. If you're a compulsive eater and see food and eating as your solution or only friend, you will *never* rid yourself of your problem. If you continue to think: "I want to lose this weight quickly so that I can eat as much as I like again", you've already lost the fight against overweight. Only when you realise that food and eating are too important to you, and that you're inclined to eat in response to emotional, physical, social or circumstantial prompts instead of when you're truly hungry, will you be on the road to recovery. This is because you realise you have a problem and need the help of a dietician and/or psychologist until you reach the point where you can say to yourself: "I can think of a hundred things I'd rather do than eat, because I'm full." The suggestions in the first part of this book will also help you get to this point, if you apply them, one by one, to your life.

> **A compulsive eater misuses food;**
> ◆ **someone who eats according to his or her needs** ◆
> **eats like a gourmet and appreciates food.**

At some point, you're going to have to give up the love of food and eating. Eating is not a good hobby for the following reasons:

- ◆ If you eat too much, you end up fat.
- ◆ If you eat too much, you'll feel guilty. This means you'll end up hating yourself, or eating even more because – you reason – you've already overdone it, so you may as well make a good job of it.
- ◆ Overeating doesn't give you the sense of achievement you experience when you've made a dress or a table, had a long chat with a friend, or had a good workout.
- ◆ You're actually supposed to eat only when you're hungry, and only until you're satisfied, not to pass the time!

So, rather find other hobbies that will distract you from food and eating, thereby freeing you from compulsive eating, helping you to lose weight and to stay slim – *permanently*.

The last word on behaviour: Make an effort!

Even if you remember nothing else you've read in this book, we'd like you to remember this: *You have to start making changes.* Most fad diets try to convince you that you can lose weight without any effort on your part. We're sure you've read or heard advertisements for slimming products or diets that promise: "Lose 5 kg in one week, without eating less or exercising more." This is the same as an advertisement that claims: "You can get *very* rich, without working or saving!" No one would believe this statement, yet they're prepared to accept, without question, that they can lose weight without making any effort.

If you accept the following, you will begin to see results
- One way to lose weight is to *eat less*. This method has been with us the longest, and is the most logical way to lose weight, yet countless people will do anything in their power not to have to eat less.
- Another way of losing weight is to *eat less often*. In other words, eat every five hours, not every hour or two.
- The method we recommend for losing weight is to *eat lower-fat, low-GI foods*, because eating fat will put on fat and low-GI foods keep you full for longer, doing away with the need to eat every hour or two.
- In addition, *becoming more active* increases your metabolic rate (the rate at which your body burns food) as well as giving you a sense of wellbeing.
- Lastly, by combining all four strategies, you're bound to be successful in your quest to lose weight.

All the worthwhile things in life require effort on our part if they are to be attained. It's unrealistic to expect to lose weight if you continue to eat the same way you've been eating for the past ten years. Remember: no "get rich quick" or "get thin quick" scheme works. The sooner you realise this, the sooner you'll begin to lose weight – and keep it off.

So, don't wait for the ideal moment to start – begin today
Some examples
- If you're going out for pizza tonight, order a smaller one than usual, or stop eating when you're full and take the rest home for breakfast tomorrow.
- If you're invited to tea, choose a few eats only, or – if you find it too difficult to resist all the delicious food – eat half portions and then compensate at the next meal.
- Try eating smaller portions, off a smaller plate. Smaller portions

look meagre on a big plate, but fill a smaller plate and give the illusion of more food.

◆ Try to eat slowly. It takes 20 minutes for your brain to register that you've eaten enough. If you stretch your meal over at least 20 minutes, you'll give your body a chance to tell you when you're full so you can stop eating when you're satiated, and not necessarily when the plate is empty.

◆ Tell yourself that you don't have to finish everything on your plate; it is permissible to leave food on your plate.

◆ Start using less oil in food preparation.

◆ Try to eat out less and to order fewer take-away meals. Most of these meals are too large and contain much more fat than meals cooked at home.

◆ Don't eat more than one main meal a day.

◆ Try to cut down on how much you eat, in every situation.

◆ Try to eat only three meals a day and to "fast" between meals (you may have something to drink and a small snack).

◆ Try to consume less alcohol, as it contains almost as many kilojoules as fat, whereas carbohydrates and protein only contain half the quantity of kilojoules.

◆ Don't pop things into your mouth while you're cooking or clearing the table. Make a point of eating at table only, off a plate, and using a knife and fork or spoon.

◆ Try to eat fewer sweets, chocolates, cakes and desserts. Usually, we eat them because they're delicious, not because we're hungry.

◆ Try to compensate as much as possible.

◆ Try to avoid eating in response to circumstances or emotions.

◆ Give up food as a hobby and develop as many non-food hobbies as possible.

◆ Find other activities that interest you and are as much fun as eating.

◆ Write down everything you eat; this often makes you realise just where you are making mistakes, in the same way as writing down all you spend makes you realise why your money runs out so quickly.

◆ Change your goal from wanting to lose weight to wanting to change from poor eating habits to normal, healthy eating behaviour.

◆ Get rid of your obsession with the scale and try to weigh yourself no more than once a week. Even better, learn to assess your weight loss, weight gain or stability by the way your clothes fit.

◆ Relearn eating in response to your body's signal that you're hungry, not in response to negative emotions or situations. Learn to listen to your body telling you when you're satisfied and should stop eating.

Begin today with a few of these suggestions and you'll be surprised at the positive impact small changes will have on your weight loss and on your life as a whole. Enlist the help of a dietician, who will give you many more tips for losing weight and maintaining the weight loss.

The last word: fad diets

It's an unfortunate fact that most people gain weight over an extended period, and that it will require an extended period to lose it. This is a fact of life many overweight people find very hard to accept. Most people gain weight, without noticing it, over a number of years. Take, for example, weight gained over the holidays. At Christmas, you gain 2 kg but *don't* lose it in January by eating less to get back to your pre-holiday weight. Then you gain another kilogram over Easter and another two in the July holidays. By the September break, you're glad that you've only gained 1 kg, but you've actually gained 6 kg over the period since Christmas. If you keep on doing this for five years, you will be 30 kg overweight. It's impossible, and unhealthy, to lose the weight you've gained over five years by following a fad diet for three months. It is possible, however, to lose this weight over a period of 9 to 12 months, following a balanced diet. And to lose the weight you gained over five years in one year is a bonus indeed!

◆ **Weight gain is gradual,
so weight loss must also be gradual.** ◆

A fad diet is merely a temporary measure. The question you have to ask yourself before you start any diet is whether you will be able to eat in this new way for the rest of your life, or, to put it differently, what your eating pattern will be once you've finished the diet. Does the diet *really* address your problem? Will it help to keep off the weight, even over the holidays, so that you don't regain all that "holiday weight" over the next five years?

In our experience, clients who regularly follow fad diets find that, having eaten only soup or grapes (i.e. no carbohydrates) for three months, they're now so starved of normal food that they end up consuming all the foods forbidden on the fad diet as though they're about to disappear forever. The result is that they end up weighing the same as they did before going on the diet – or even more! To achieve permanent weight loss you have to develop a long-term perspective.

 **Don't ask: "How am I going to lose this weight?"
Rather ask: "How long am I going to stay slim?"**

Let's look at an analogy. Say you earn R5 000 a month, but spend R6 000 a month. If you were to continue spending R1 000 more than you earn every month, your bank account would be overdrawn by R10 000 within ten months. To remedy this, you would do a few sums and find ways to cut down your expenses to R5 000.

This is the same as suddenly discovering that you've gained a lot of weight. Spending R1 000 less every month will ensure that you break even every month, but it will not help to pay off your debt. This is analogous to a maintenance diet; you "break even", but don't lose weight.

To pay off the debt, you'd have to cut your monthly expenses even more, say by R500 or R1 000, so that your total expenditure is no more than R4 500 or even R4 000. For a while this will be difficult, but not half as difficult as it is to cut your expenses by half, to R3 000 a month, which would be comparable to going on a fad diet. You've over-indulged for the past ten months, so you should be able to make do if you cut your expenditure by a little over R1 000 a month. This is an analogy for the balanced slimming diet. Once you've paid off your debt, you will also make sure that your monthly expenses do not exceed R5 000, so that you don't end up with the same debt again in six months' time. This is the analogy for a balanced maintenance diet. Alternatively, you could secure another income (or, in terms of the analogy, become more active) so that you can spend R6 000 a month without getting into debt (or picking up weight). Can you see the similarity between the two scenarios?

It always amazes us that intelligent people, who would only hire the best person for a given job, will resort to all sorts of unqualified people and means when it comes to their health or to weight loss, instead of seeking out the help of the best-qualified person. Surely you wouldn't take your sick dog to the dentist, or your broken-down car to a beautician, or consult an undertaker when you want to paint your house? Of course you wouldn't. Maybe you think we're off our heads even to suggest such things, yet that is exactly what people do! Every day, people respond to advertisements for losing weight in magazines, on trees or street poles, or on cars. They turn to books, magazines, doctors, pharmacists, beauticians, and even totally unqualified people for advice, and follow a fad diet, drink milkshakes, take tablets, wear sweat suits, and adopt many other crutches in their quest to lose weight. Although many of the people mentioned above are well qualified to do a wide variety of things, they are totally unqualified to give you dietary advice.

 A dietician is the person best qualified to give you dietary advice.

When it comes to diet-related problems, including weight loss, consult a registered dietician who will help you get to the root of your weight or diet-related problem and thus enable you to cope with it for the rest of your life. For a list of dieticians who use the Glycemic Index in their treatment of patients, visit the GIFSA (Glycemic Index Foundation of South Africa) website at www.gifoundation.com.

These are some of the fad diets available today.

1. High-protein, low-carbohydrate diets

Any diet that advises you to check your urine for ketones or restricts the intake of carbohydrates (starch, dried beans, peas and lentils, fruit, certain vegetables, dairy products and sweet things) is unbalanced and impossible to follow for any length of time. *Such an eating pattern would also be very difficult to follow for the rest of your life.*

Carbohydrates are our bodies' main source of energy (fuel), and if there isn't enough fuel available at any one time, our bodies will burn body proteins and fats. The consequences are:

- Lean body mass (muscle) loss, which lowers your metabolic rate.
- Increased production of ketones, resulting in a condition known as keto-acidosis. If left untreated, this may result in coma and possibly death.
- Kidney damage may also result, as a high-protein diet places a huge burden on the kidneys.
- These diets are also very expensive.
- Tiredness and lack of energy. This type of diet usually advises you not to exercise as you won't have the energy to do so. This, in turn, results in further lean body mass loss, which further reduces the basal metabolic rate.
- Those who follow this type of diet again and again, with the concomitant weight gain each time, will end up with a much larger percentage of body fat and increasingly less lean body mass.
- Eating more than 80 g protein (350 g meat, fish, chicken or cheese) a day increases your risk for osteoporosis. This is because proteins are made up of amino acids, which have to be neutralised by the body. The body does this by drawing alkaline calcium out of the bones. In addition, this type of diet is usually very low in calcium, which increases your chances of developing osteoporosis and/or arthritis, if followed for any length of time. High intakes of meat, fish and chicken and low intakes of starch and dairy products often lead to high purine levels, which predispose to gout.

Lastly, consider this: A meal of 120 g or more of meat, fish, chicken or cheese, with no starch and only one portion of vegetables or salad, can be replaced by a meal consisting of 30 g to 60 g of meat, fish, chicken or cheese, one to two portions of low-GI starch, and vegetables or salad. You get the same kilojoules (calories), with less fat – even the leanest meat and chicken contain some fat – whereas most pure starches are fat-free. This last meal is better balanced, gives you more energy, and is easy to follow for the rest of your life!

Fat is fattening; carbohydrates aren't, but watch your portions.

2. High-protein, high-fat diets

Most of these diets permit the consumption of huge quantities of protein such as meat, fish, chicken, cheese, eggs, etc. as well as unlimited quantities of fat. They advocate using cream in coffee or tea, rather than milk, and you're not required to remove the visible fat off bacon, chops, etc.

At first glance this seems wonderful, but again it is not an ideal diet to follow.

◆ In the long run, you'll get tired of eating bacon and eggs, without toast, for breakfast every morning; of eating cheese without bread; or meat, fish and chicken without any rice, potatoes or other starch.

◆ In addition, this type of high-protein, high-fat eating can lead to all sorts of lifestyle diseases, such as diabetes, high blood pressure, hyperlidemia (high cholesterol and/or high triglyceride levels), hyperinsulinaemia, insulin resistance, etc.

◆ Because carbohydrates initiate an insulin response in the body and because insulin is a fat storer, it may seem that avoiding carbohydrates is the best course of action. Not so! Both fat and protein also elicit an insulin response, and have a delayed effect on blood glucose levels. Low-GI carbohydrates have only a limited effect on blood glucose levels, and even high-GI carbohydrates have a minor effect on blood glucose levels, after exercise. Eating the right kind of carbohydrate, therefore, will keep insulin levels within normal ranges.

◆ All the disadvantages of the high-protein, low-carbohydrate diet apply here as well.

3. Mono food diets

You probably know these diets all too well: the soup diet, for example, or the pineapple diet, the grape diet, the banana diet, the fruit and nut diet, etc. These diets are not ideal for the following reasons.

◆ It is only a matter of time before you get thoroughly bored with eating only one type of food and it certainly isn't a diet you could follow for the rest of your life.

◆ This type of diet doesn't address the bad eating habits that led to your weight gain, and certainly doesn't teach you how to eat correctly.

◆ A mono food diet is completely unbalanced, which means you will pick up deficiencies of one nutrient or another in the long run. For example, if dairy products are excluded, you may develop osteoporosis and arthritis.

◆ Most mono food diets are also too low in protein. This means that the body doesn't have enough raw materials to build body tissues, which in turn can lead to a loss of lean body mass. As you are aware by now, this lowers the metabolic rate, especially if it's combined with very low kilojoule intakes, as is normally the case.

◆ Such a diet can even be too high in fat; for example, if you end up eating big bags of nuts on the fruit and nut diet.

4. Very low kilojoule diets

The less you eat, the quicker you will lose weight, right? Wrong! Here's why:

◆ Diets that contain less than 4 200 kJ (1 000 calories) don't provide enough energy for the body to carry out normal daily functions, let alone enough energy for sport or exercise.

◆ In addition, your body sees this drastic reduction in energy intake as a threat (starvation) and can lower its metabolic rate by as much as 45% in response! This is a protective mechanism the body adopts if it perceives that there are months of food shortage ahead. It also hangs on to as much fat as possible, to ensure that you will survive the starvation period. Not exactly what you had in mind!

◆ It's easier for the body to convert protein to energy, than to use fat. As a result, most of the weight lost will be lean body mass (muscle), which means your metabolic rate will decrease as the weight is lost. This effect is exaggerated if you don't exercise. The result is that you lose precious lean body mass and water, not the body fat you intended losing. As soon as you start eating "normally" again, you start retaining water; you could even develop a persistent water retention problem.

◆ While you're on a very low kilojoule diet you won't feel very well and could suffer from dizziness, lack of energy, inability to concentrate, tiredness, sleepiness, etc.

So, for effective weight loss, you have to "fool" your body into thinking that everything is still okay. If you reduce your energy intake by no more than 2 000 kJ to 4 000 kJ (500 to 1 000 calories) a day, your body will be willing to lose the excess body fat.

5. Food combining

One school of thought, which is against food combining, believes that if proteins and carbohydrates are eaten together, weight loss is not possible. The reason people lose weight on these diets is that they simply eat much less, not because protein and starch cannot be eaten together.

For optimal control of blood glucose levels, sustained energy and absence of hunger, a meal containing low-GI carbohydrate, a little protein and a little fat is ideal. Protein and fat help to control glucose absorption by delaying gastric emptying. This aids in weight loss as blood glucose levels are kept constant. In light of the fact that most overweight people have problems controlling blood glucose levels, it can only be of benefit to combine protein and carbohydrate in every meal.

Dairy products are often limited as well on food-combining diets. This makes for an unbalanced diet, as everyone, including adults, needs a certain amount of calcium for normal muscle function and sound bone structure.

And, as any dietician can tell you, it's impossible to separate carbohydrates and proteins completely as they come together naturally in food. Most vegetables and starches contain a little protein, and protein sources such as milk, yoghurt and legumes (dried beans, peas and lentils) and nuts (which also contain a lot of fat), contain equal quantities of starch and protein. So eating salad with fish, or even yoghurt by itself, involves combining carbohydrate and protein. Not quite what these diets advocate.

6. Very low fat or fat-free diets

The internationally accepted definitions for fat-free and low-fat foods are as follows:

Fat-free: less than, or equal to, 0,5 g fat per 100 g food

Low-fat: less than, or equal to, 3 g fat per 100 g food

Our recommendation is to follow a *lower*-fat diet, rather than a fat-free or low-fat diet. The reason for this is that the quantities of essential fatty acids in fat-containing foods would be too low on a fat-free or low-fat diet. In addition, it is very difficult to eat fat-free or low-fat foods for the rest of your life; in fact, too little fat can actually *prevent* fat loss!

Let us explain. If you wish to eat only those foods that contain 3 g or less fat per 100 g, you would only be allowed to eat white fish and skinned chicken breasts, as well as all fruit and vegetables. Eggs would not be permitted, neither would red meat, and only fat-free cottage cheese would be allowed. In addition, you may only use skimmed milk. While you may be able to follow such a diet for some time, it would require great discipline to do so for the rest of your life.

Following a very low fat diet – i.e. less than 25% of your total kilojoule intake – means you would have to eat a diet very high in carbohydrates. As long as the carbohydrates you eat are low Glycemic Index (GI), this diet could work for you. If you end up eating mostly high-GI carbohydrates, however, you put yourself at risk of developing blood glucose control problems and maybe even diabetes. As you will learn in the next section, blood glucose control is vital for successful weight loss.

As mentioned earlier, a shortage of fat in the diet might even prevent weight loss. The reasons for this are:

◆ Mono-unsaturated fats play a critical role in controlling the secretion of insulin, the fat-storing hormone, because they slow the rate at which carbohydrates are digested and released into the bloodstream. Ironically, this also enables the body to burn fat stores more efficiently, as a source of energy. So a little fat is needed every day to ensure that fat is effectively used as a source of energy.

◆ By slowing down the digestion and absorption of carbohydrates, fats can actually help with satiety, making you feel full for longer and in this way helping you with your weight loss programme.

But remember that fat always makes fat, no matter how "good" it is. For this reason, portion control is vital; we recommend about three to six portions of fat a day. The exact quantity will depend on each individual, male or female, your level of activity, and whether you want to lose or maintain weight. The recommended quantity of fat should be spread out throughout the day, and some fat should be included in every meal.

A balanced diet should contain no less than 25% – 30% fat, which amounts to about 30 g fat per 4 200 kJ. If you eat mainly foods that contain 3 g fat per 100 g – or at least those that contain no more than 3 g – 10 g fat per 100 g – you will easily stay within the fat allowance.

7. Milkshakes/meal replacements

Did you know that one of these slimming shakes contains as many kilojoules as a breakfast or a light meal? Speaking for ourselves, we'd far rather eat three balanced meals a day than replace one, two or all three meals with a slimming shake. In the long run, drinking milk-shakes instead of eating meals can be rather expensive, and again it doesn't address your original bad eating habits. And be honest: Could you drink them for the rest of your life? One of our patients decided to replace one meal a day with a slimming shake to speed up her weight loss. To her consternation, she actually *gained* weight in that week, and she vowed never to try a milkshake diet again!

8. Tablets and tonics

Almost every week we're bombarded with advertisements for slim-ming pills and tonics that appear to be the wonder cure for over-weight people. They promise all sorts of benefits, such as increasing your metabolic rate, burning body fat, "trapping" dietary fat to pre-vent the body from absorbing it, suppressing your appetite, and so on. They promise great weight loss without you having to change your eating habits or increase how much you exercise, and all with-in a short space of time.

Let's look at some of these slimming pills and tonics.

◆ *Those that increase metabolic rate*: These tablets and tonics con-tain large quantities of caffeine and/or ephedrine. While both substances increase your metabolic rate, they do so at a price. You become so hyperactive that you experience heart palpita-tions and feel shaky most of the time, which has a negative impact on your work and sleep.

◆ *Those that burn fat*: There's no such thing as a substance that can burn fat. To lose body fat, you have to eat less (especially fat) and be more active, so that your body uses up more kilojoules.

◆ *Fat trappers*: Some products on the market do "trap" fat, but unfortunately they absorb all the good fats (mono- and polyunsaturated fats), and this could result in dry skin, high cholesterol levels, arthritis, hyperactivity and even being overweight. In addition, for these capsules/tablets to be effective when eating a high-fat meal, you'd have to take eight capsules at a time. This is *not* the kind of habit anyone should be nurturing. When dietary fat is lost to the body in this way, the fat-soluble vitamins don't get absorbed either. And this could lead to a whole host of other deficiency problems.

◆ *Appetite suppressants*: If you follow our low-GI eating plan (see pages 156 – 165), exercise regularly and learn to listen to your body's hunger and satiety signals, you won't need any appetite suppressants. Vegetables are the most filling foods available, so include them at every meal, together with water. (Contrary to popular belief, water doesn't dilute gastric juices.)

9. Fasting before and after exercise

This diet is based on the incorrect belief that fat burning will be optimised if no food is consumed before exercising, because food stimulates the release of insulin, which is a fat storer. Research has shown, to the contrary, that eating low-GI carbohydrates 1 – 2 hours before exercising actually enhances sporting performance and endurance. (See page 90).

This diet also recommends that no food or drink, except water, be taken for 1 – 2 hours after exercise. This advice is not only incorrect, but could be harmful. Research has shown that higher-GI foods or drinks must be consumed within half an hour of exercising, in order to avoid post-exercise low blood sugar levels and having to drag yourself around all day, feeling debilitated, because your energy level is low.

10. Injections

Many fad diets are accompanied by weekly injections, which are supposed to stimulate your body to burn fat. The injections may also contain vitamins, as most of these diets are totally unbalanced and lacking in vitamins. In most cases, any weight loss is due to the restricted food intake, not the injections. As we've mentioned before, this kind of weight loss comes from precious lean body mass loss or water loss, not the excess body fat you're trying to get rid of.

Most of our patients who've followed such a diet and had the injections, have reported that once they stopped the diet and started eating normally again, they regained all the lost weight – and more. Research tells us that a lot of weight can be lost in a short space of time on a fad diet, but that this weight loss is very rarely permanent. In contrast, a sensible eating plan, together with positive changes in eating habits and regular exercise, results in more permanent weight loss, although it does take a little longer.

Summary

Don't be duped by the wonderful results promised by fad diets. Most of the weight lost on these diets comes from lean (muscle) body mass, with resultant lowering of the basal metabolic rate. A lot of the weight loss is also water loss, and very little body fat is lost. For this reason, people who are always on diet, end up becoming fatter and fatter.

In the next section we will give you more information about our low-GI, lower-fat eating plan that you can follow for the rest of your life.

Low-GI, lower-fat eating

What should you eat?

Introduction

Firstly, this is not a diet but a nutritional (eating) plan – for your entire life. It's a way of living that will bring you a longer life packed with vitality, wellness and optimal health. Unfortunately, there's no such thing as a quick fix. But after you've stuck to your eating plan for a while, the positive results you see should be well worth the small effort of eating the low Glycemic Index (GI), lower fat way most of the time.

The good news is that after only a few days of eating the low Glycemic Index (GI), lower fat way, your blood sugar and insulin levels will be within the normal metabolic range, and within two weeks you will no longer experience chronic hunger, cravings and feelings of deprivation. This means that you'll feel a marked improvement in mental focus, exercise endurance, strength, optimal health, muscularity and leanness.

The low-GI, lower-fat eating plan isn't something we've dreamt up; it's based on years of experience in our dietetic practices. It also has a firm base in worldwide research over the last twenty years and is so logical that we cannot believe we didn't think of it before.

What makes you fat?

Put very simply, it's mostly a combination of too many refined or high-GI carbohydrates, such as biscuits, crackers and white bread, too much visible and hidden fat (especially of the wrong kind), not enough exercise, and eating for the wrong reasons. Add uncontrollable cravings for these refined or high-GI carbohydrates, for whatever reason, and you have a recipe for disaster.

The life-long low-GI, lower-fat nutritional plan is suitable for *everyone*, including those suffering from diabetes (Types 1 and 2), heart disease, hypertension (high blood pressure), arthritis, hyperinsulinaemia (high insulin levels in the blood), hypoglycemia, chronic candida infections, polycystic ovarian syndrome (PCOS), attention deficit hyperactivity syndrome (ADHD) and insulin resistance. It is eminently suitable for the whole family, which means no extra preparation or isolation from the rest of the family as you force down the "diet food", while the rest of them enjoy a tasty meal.

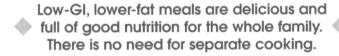

Low-GI, lower-fat meals are delicious and full of good nutrition for the whole family. There is no need for separate cooking.

As explained in the previous section, carbohydrates are not the enemy many slimmers have been brainwashed into thinking they are. It is true that overindulgence in too many of the wrong carbohydrates, at the wrong time, can cause problems such as weight gain, or falling asleep during board meetings, or even compromising athletic performance, but it's equally true that the right carbohydrates, at the right time and in the right quantities, are the key to optimising your body's functioning and your performance. It's just a matter of knowing what to look for in a carbohydrate, which carbohydrate to eat when, and how much of it to eat.

The reason carbohydrates have gained such a poor reputation is that many pure carbohydrate foods, such as potatoes and most breads, can dramatically affect your blood glucose levels when eaten on their own. This results in a surge of insulin being secreted, and this in turn stimulates the secretion of the fat storage enzyme, lipoprotein lipase (LPL). The nett effect is an increase in your fat stores with resultant weight gain.

Regulating blood insulin levels is thus of vital importance in successful weight loss and keeping your body in top form. In fact, when insulin levels are out of kilter, and particularly when there is hyperinsulinaemia, you could be plagued with recurrent feelings of hunger and cravings, as well as mood swings, lethargy, obesity, poor athletic performance, loss of endurance, training failures, insulin resistance and even a shortened life span. Many chronic diseases, including diabetes, heart disease, cancer, a suppressed immune system, chronic candida infections, or polycystic ovarian syndrome (PCOS) may also result.

The secret is to work out the effect a particular carbohydrate food will have on your blood glucose levels. Fortunately for all of us, the Glycemic Index of many carbohydrate foods has already been determined worldwide, and gives us an easy way of deciding the value of a specific carbohydrate. To make your life easier, we've rated a whole range of common carbohydrate foods in this book, both in alphabetical order (pages 229 – 246) and according to food groups (pages 219 – 228). For a detailed explanation of the Glycemic Index and how it is tested, please read pages 79 to 85.

In brief, the Glycemic Index (GI) refers to the relative degree to which the concentration of blood glucose rises after consumption of a food. It doesn't indicate the actual level of sugar in the blood; instead, it shows the relative percentage of the *effect* of the food on blood glucose levels compared with the effect of pure glucose. Some of what you're about to learn will contradict what you probably thought about these foods, and will certainly surprise you. So read on to see which carbohydrates are good for weight loss and good health, and which carbohydrates can be detrimental to your health and hinder weight loss.

Fats, on the other hand, do have to be restricted, but certainly not as strictly as has been advocated in the last decade. More recent research has shown that very low fat intakes are detrimental to body functioning, and that a "lower" fat intake is the most desirable for sustained weight loss. In fact, you need to consume a small quantity of good-quality fats on a regular basis in order to lose weight, as explained in the section on fad diets (page 56). Read on to find out how to "fat-proof" your meals with the right quantity and type of fat.

We've compiled two questionnaires for you to complete in this section, so that you can find out what the average GI of your meals comes to, and how high your fat intake is.

Chapter 4

The Glycemic Index (GI)

Glycemic Index Questionnaire

What is the overall GI of your diet?

To find out how high the Glycemic Index of your present diet is, complete the following questionnaire and add up your scores. Ratings are given at the end of the questionnaire.

Section A

Please complete the following questionnaire by ticking the appropriate box.

		0	1	2	3	4	5+
1.	On average, how many slices of white, brown or wholewheat bread do you eat a day (toast, sandwiches, etc.)? Don't count those eaten after exercise.	0	1	2	3	4	5+
2.	In a week, how many times do you eat cooked porridge? Don't count that eaten after exercise.	0	1	2	3	4	5+
3.	In a week, how many times do you eat refined cereals (Rice Krispies, cornflakes, etc.)? Don't count those eaten after exercise.	0	1	2	3	4	5+
4.	In a week, how many times do you eat scones/crumpets/muffins/rusks? Don't count those eaten after exercise.	0	1	2	3	4	5+
5.	In a week, how many times do you eat sweet biscuits and cakes? Don't count those eaten after exercise.	0	1	2	3	4	5+
6.	In a week, how many cans (340 ml) of fizzy cooldrinks (Coke, Fanta, Sprite, etc.) do you drink? (If you drink from a bigger bottle poured into glasses, estimate how many cans this would be equal to.)	0	1	2	3	4	5+
7.	On an average day, how many sweets do you eat? (Jelly babies, toffees, liquorice allsorts, marshmallows, etc.) Don't count those eaten after exercise.	0	1	2	3	4	5+

8.	In a week, how often do you eat chocolate bars, chocolate slabs or fudge? Don't count those eaten after exercise.	0	1	2	3	4	5+
9.	How many times a week do you have an instant or packet soup? Don't count those eaten after exercise.	0	1	2	3	4	5+
10.	How many times a week do you eat potatoes (boiled, baked, wedges, chips, mashed; excluding baby potatoes with skin). Don't count those eaten after exercise.	0	1	2	3	4	5+
11.	How many sports drinks/ energy drinks (500 ml) do you drink every week? Don't count those drunk after exercise.	0	1	2	3	4	5+
12.	How many times a week do you eat yellow pumpkin and squashes? Don't count those eaten after exercise.	0	1	2	3	4	5+
13.	How many times a week do you eat melons (spanspek, watermelon, sweet melon, etc.)? Don't count those eaten after exercise.	0	1	2	3	4	5+
14.	How many rolls (white and brown) do you eat a week? Don't count those eaten after exercise.	0	1	2	3	4	5+

Now add up all your ticked numbers to give your total.

Total A _____

Section B

Please tick the block containing the answer that fits best.

1.	How many portions of cooked vegetables do you eat a week?	0	1	2	3	4	5+
	B1 score	6	5	4	3	2	1
2.	How many times a week do you eat raw vegetables or salads?	0	1	2	3	4	5+
	B2 score	6	5	4	3	2	1
3.	How often do you eat sweet potatoes?	more than twice a week	twice per week	once per week	once per month	occasionally	never
	B3 score	1	1	2	3	4	5
4.	How often do you eat pearled barley or pearled wheat (stampkoring/ wheat rice) as a starch with your dinner?	more than twice a week	twice per week	once per week	once per month	occasionally	never
	B4 score	0	1	2	3	4	5
5.	How often do you eat basmati or Tastic rice?	more than twice a week	twice per week	once per week	once per month	occasionally	never
	B5 score	0	1	2	3	4	5
6.	How many times a week do you eat yoghurt (fruit or plain)?	six times per week	five times per week	four times per week	two or three times a week	once per week	never
	B6 score	0	1	2	3	4	5
7.	How many times a week do you eat baked beans?	five times per week	four times per week	three times per week	twice per week	once per week	never
	B7 score	0	1	2	3	4	5

8.	How many pieces of deciduous and citrus fruit do you eat every day? (Apples, pears, apricots, peaches, nectarines, grapes, kiwifruit, cherries, plums, oranges, naartjies, grapefruit, etc.)	five	four	three	two	one	none
	B8 score	0	1	2	3	4	5
9.	How many pieces of tropical fruit do you eat every day? (Bananas, pawpaw, mangoes, litchis, pineapple, etc.) Don't count those eaten after exercise.	five	four	three	two	one	none
	B9 score	3	3	2	2	1	0
10.	How many times a week do you eat lentils?	five times per week	four times per week	three times per week	twice per week	once per week	never
	B10 score	0	1	2	3	4	5
11.	How many times a week do you eat cooked dried beans or split peas (in soups, stews, casseroles, stir-fries)?	five times per week	four times per week	three times per week	twice per week	once per week	never
	B11 score	0	1	2	3	4	5
12.	How many times a week do you use oats, oat bran or split lentils in your meals?	never	once a week	twice a week	three times a week	four times a week	five or more times a week
	B12 score	5	4	3	2	1	0
13.	How many slices of Cape Seed Loaf or wheat-free rye bread do you eat a week?	five or more slices	four	three	two	one	none
	B13 score	0	1	2	3	4	5

14.	How many times a week do you eat good-quality pasta (made from durum wheat)?	five or more times per week	four times per week	three times per week	twice per week	once per week	never
	B14 score	0	1	2	3	4	5

Now add up your scores under each block ticked to give your total.

Total B _____

Add the total from Section A to your total from Section B.

Grand total _____

Scoring
55 or under
Well done! Your intake is mainly from low-GI foods. If you do eat higher-GI foods, you do so after exercise, which is as it should be. You've obviously had some training in the Glycemic Index and know how to put it into practice.

Keep it up!

56 – 69
You've obviously heard of the Glycemic Index, but are unsure how to put it into practice. You need to read the next section carefully so that you can grasp the concept of the Glycemic Index fully. Once you really understand it, it will be easy to put into practice.

70 and over
Oh dear! You're eating a typical high-GI diet, so common in our modern world of eating on the run. High-GI meals result in high insulin levels, and elevated insulin levels can, over time, do quite a lot of damage to your body, including preventing weight loss. It is important that you learn about the Glycemic Index and how to choose low-GI foods. You need to stop eating all those refined carbohydrates and start introducing lower-GI starches, vegetables, fruits and legumes (dried beans, peas and lentils) into your meals on a daily basis.

Read on …

What Is the Glycemic Index (GI)?

Before we can explain the Glycemic Index, we need to discuss the basics of food digestion.

When we eat carbohydrates – starches, fruit, vegetables, dairy products, legumes and sweet things – they're digested in the stomach and intestines and are then absorbed into the bloodstream in the form of glucose.

The glucose in the blood then stimulates the pancreas to produce and secrete the hormone insulin into the bloodstream. This hormone helps body cells to take up glucose from the blood, so that the cells can use it for energy.

The effect of eating is, therefore, that we increase both our blood glucose and insulin levels.

Researchers have discovered that not all carbohydrates are digested and absorbed at the same rate. This means that different carbohydrates have different effects on blood glucose and blood insulin levels.

This difference is called the Glycemic Index or GI.

Let's start by breaking up the term into its component parts:

- *Gly-*, in medical terms, stands for *glucose*
- *-aemic*, in medical terms, stands for *blood*
- *Index* means an indicator of some kind

If we put the parts of the words together, we get the meaning that the Glycemic Index is a "blood glucose indicator".

> This means that we can use the Glycemic Index (GI) as a measure, on a scale from 0 to 100, of how fast a carbohydrate-containing food is digested and absorbed. It gives us an indication of the rate at which the food affects blood glucose levels after ingestion of the carbohydrate-containing food.

Glucose is assigned a numerical value of 100 because it is absorbed into the bloodstream almost immediately, providing a sharp, quick rise in blood glucose levels. All other carbohydrate foods are compared to this as the standard.

In some research studies, white bread is used as the standard. If bread is used, the Glycemic Index of glucose must be higher than that for bread and as a result all the values will be higher. For example, the GI of cornflakes is 84 when tested against glucose, whereas it is 100 when tested against bread.

In South Africa, glucose is the preferred standard, since it is more practical to take glucose, not bread, as 100; bread actually causes a 70% rise in blood glucose levels, when compared to glucose.

When consulting different Glycemic Index tables, however, it is important to check whether the values have been determined using bread or glucose as the reference food, otherwise you could get confused. And to make matters even more confusing, many authors mix up the two without realising it!

So be very careful when you look up GI values in tables. Always check which food has been used as the reference food: glucose or bread. To convert a GI with bread as the reference food, simply multiply the value by 0,7. To convert from glucose to bread as the reference food, multiply by 1,43.

And if you're still not sure, visit the website of the Glycemic Index Foundation of South Africa (GIFSA) at www.gifoundation.com to get reliable information on the Glycemic Index of different foods.

Throughout this book, we'll be referring to GI values using glucose as the reference food.

GI conversion factors for different reference foods
◆ Glucose to bread x 1,43
◆ Bread to glucose x 0,7

Carbohydrate foods with GI values nearer 100 (high-GI foods) are digested and absorbed faster than those carbohydrate foods with GI values of 55 and below (low-GI foods). Standard South African bread (including white and brown bread), for example, has a GI of between 72 and 81 and butter beans have a GI of 31. This means that the bread would provide a sharper, quicker rise in blood glucose levels than the butter beans.

All high-GI foods are digested and absorbed very quickly, providing a steep rise in blood glucose levels. See graph opposite.

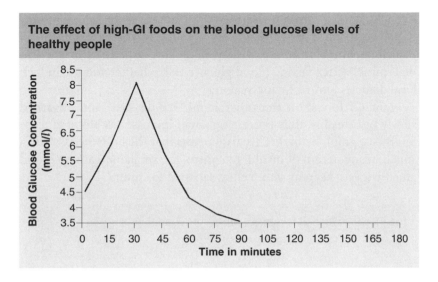

The effect of high-GI foods on the blood glucose levels of healthy people

In an effort to keep blood glucose levels as near to normal as possible, the body will sensitise the pancreas to produce a surge of insulin to take care of the huge increase in blood glucose levels. This extra insulin then rapidly lowers blood glucose levels, creating a "witch's hat" type of graph. Blood glucose levels surge up the one side of the "witch's hat", then come screaming down the other side, which is also very aptly referred to as "the blood sugar roller coaster"!

If this surge in glucose levels is repeated several times a day, the pancreas will eventually overproduce insulin and the consequent drop in blood glucose levels will result in reactive hypoglycaemia. If someone continues to eat high-GI foods most of the time, without food combining or eating them after exercise, he or she is at risk of developing Impaired Glucose Tolerance (IGT), or pre-diabetes – and, eventually, Type 2 diabetes – because the insulin stores of the pancreas have become depleted. This can also lead to hyperinsulinaemia, insulin resistance, hypertension (high blood pressure) and overweight. (See page 85 for information on hyperinsulinaemia and insulin resistance.)

Once someone has become diabetic, however, high-GI foods will no longer cause a "witch's hat" type of curve on the graph. Instead, blood glucose levels will remain elevated for long periods, which is very detrimental to the body. Should you suspect that you have hypoglycaemia or diabetes, refer to the GIFSA website (www.gifoundation.com) for a list of dieticians who follow the Glycemic Index principles. You should also visit your doctor so that he or she can determine, with a fasting blood glucose test, whether you do, in fact, have diabetes and/or hypoglycaemia.

Low-GI foods, on the other hand, are digested and absorbed slowly but steadily, thus producing small increases in blood glucose levels (see graph below). This also means that the body needs only a small, steady stream of insulin to control the small increases in blood glucose levels, keeping you feeling satisfied for hours.

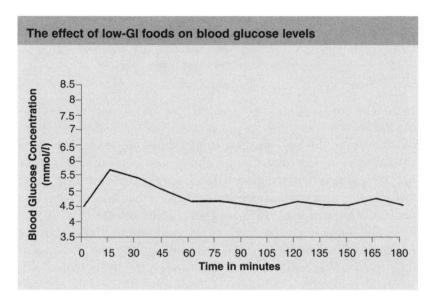

From these graphs, it now becomes clear that the carbohydrate supplied by bread would only provide fuel for body cells for less than one hour, whereas butter beans would provide a smaller, but steady, trickle of fuel for $2^1/_2 - 3$ hours. A meal containing butter beans, therefore, would keep you feeling full for much longer than a meal based on bread. In addition, *the body would have to secrete much less insulin* to deal with the carbohydrate from butter beans, than it would for the large quantity of carbohydrate dumped into the bloodstream by bread.

Physiologically speaking, the lower-GI carbohydrate foods are much less taxing on the body, and this can help prevent hypoglycaemia, IGT, Type 2 diabetes, hyperinsulinaemia, insulin resistance, hypertension and overweight.

Based on the Glycemic Index of each carbohydrate-containing food, carbohydrates are divided into three broad categories:

◆ Carbohydrate foods with a GI value of 55 and under are regarded as low-GI foods.

◆ Carbohydrate foods with GI values of between 56 and 69 are regarded as intermediate-GI foods.

◆ All carbohydrate foods with GI values of 70 and over are regarded as high-GI foods.

It is not imperative, however, to know the exact GI value of every food. Even we, who work with the Glycemic Index every day, don't know the exact GI value of every single carbohydrate-containing food. To learn all those values would be far too tedious and time-consuming. It's much better to *understand the concept* of the Glycemic Index and to be able to identify those foods that are absorbed slowly over a longer period of time, i.e. the low-GI foods, and those that are dumped into the blood stream as a surge of glucose, i.e. the high-GI foods.

The Glycemic Index lists at the back of this book list all the foods that have so far been tested for their GI values, in the three broad categories, without burdening you with the actual values:

Low-GI foods (listed in green)

Intermediate-GI foods (listed in orange); and

High-GI foods (listed in red).

However, should you wish to look up the exact GI value of a particular food, please visit the website of the Glycemic Index Foundation of South Africa (GIFSA) at www.gifoundation.com. GIFSA is a reliable source of information regarding the Glycemic Index of any food.

If you'd like to know the GI value of a particular food, however, and can't find it in the lists at the back of this book or in the *SA GI Guide*, available from GIFSA's website, please phone the toll-free number on the product packaging and ask the manufacturer what the GI is. If they don't know, encourage them to have the GI of the food tested. The manufacturer can then contact Liesbet at dellas@mweb.co.za or Gabi at gabist@mweb.co.za to inquire about having the GI of a product determined.

How is the Glycemic Index of a food determined?

Tests to determine the GI value of a given food are performed on real people, eating real food, and taking real blood glucose readings.

The test team

A team of testers is made up of volunteers who are all highly motivated and thoroughly trained. A team usually consists of at least eight people, but preferably twelve. People with different blood glucose control problems, as well as those without problems, are used as subjects (testers), i.e. those who have diabetes (Type 1 and Type 2, controlled by insulin, medication or diet alone), those without diabetes, those who exercise and those who don't.

The test food portion size

To ensure that all Glycemic Index testing carried out worldwide is consistent, the portion size has been standardised to 50 g available or glycemic carbohydrate in the food. This means that the portion of food tested must contain exactly 50 g of carbohydrate that is available to the body for digestion and that will affect blood glucose levels after ingestion.

For example, if apples need to be tested, each subject would have to eat about three apples weighing exactly 380 g in total, since this quantity contains exactly 50 g available or glycemic carbohydrate. If glucose were being tested, each subject would have to consume exactly 50 g of glucose, which is about 45 ml (3 T). Should fruit juice need to be tested, each tester would have to drink about 350 ml to 450 ml ($1^2/_5$ C to $1^4/_5$ C) of the juice (depending on the flavour).

As you can see, the portion size is quite large, and this is done on purpose. If a large portion of a given food results in a small rise in blood glucose levels after eating the food, we can be sure that a more normal, smaller portion will be quite safe and have only a limited impact on blood glucose levels. Also remember that the Glycemic Index is not an *absolute* value; it compares the effect of 50 g glycemic carbohydrate of a given food on blood glucose levels with the effect of 50 g glucose on the blood glucose levels *in the same person*.

The testing procedure

Before consuming the test food, the starting point is determined by taking blood glucose levels after a standard evening meal and overnight fast. The food to be tested is then eaten within 15 minutes. The blood glucose readings are taken every 15 minutes afterwards, for two to three hours. In diabetics, blood glucose readings are never taken for more than three hours and in normo-glycemic people (people who do not have blood glucose control problems), readings are never taken for more than two hours. All the readings are entered on a graph, similar to those on pages XX and XX, where blood glucose concentrations are plotted against time elapsed. The area under the graph of the test food is compared to the area under the graph of the glucose test average (the reference food is tested on three occasions) of the specific subject, and this gives us the Glycemic Index value in that specific person. This means that the numerical value obtained is a *ratio* value (test food over glucose, the reference food), and that is why it's relatively constant in *all* people. The GI of a given food is, however, the average of the GI values obtained from the eight or twelve individual subjects.

The advantages of eating the low-GI way

Research has shown that moderately high carbohydrate, lower-fat diets result in better weight loss (i.e. 50% – 55% of total energy coming from carbohydrates, 25 – 30% from fats and 15 – 20% from protein) than low-carbohydrate diets. (*Journal of the American Dietetic Association*, 2001). Lower fat intakes as opposed to no fat intakes have also been shown to be more successful for weight loss. (See explanation in the section on fad diets, page 56.) This means that moderately high carbohydrate diets with moderate fat restriction give the best long-term results. Combine this with the consumption of mainly lower GI carbohydrates and a healthy quantity of protein, and you end up with a really successful slimming formula.

1. Helps to prevent hyperinsulinaemia, insulin resistance and the Metabolic Syndrome

Continuous consumption of high-GI foods and meals means the pancreas has to pour out vast quantities of insulin continuously in order to try to maintain homeostasis of blood glucose levels or – to put it simply – to keep body fuel levels within normal ranges so it will function optimally. This results in high insulin levels in the bloodstream. The medical term for this is hyperinsulinaemia. See "Improved weight loss" (page 87) for an in-depth discussion of hyperinsulinaemia and insulin resistance.

If you haven't yet read the section explaining what the Glycemic Index is, now is the time to turn back to page 79 and come to grips with how different foods affect body fuel (blood glucose) levels.

Hyperinsulinaemia or high insulin levels result in:

◆ Stimulation of lipoprotein lipase (LPL), the enzyme that promotes fat storage
◆ Exacerbation of Attention Deficit Hyperactivity Disorder (ADHD)
◆ Impairment of sports performance resulting from insulin surges
◆ Possible reactive hypoglycaemia, which can easily progress to IGT (pre-diabetes) and eventually to Type 2 diabetes
◆ Poor glycemic control in diabetics, with the development of insulin resistance and the Metabolic Syndrome (also called Syndrome X or Insulin Resistance Syndrome), a condition present in most overweight people and in diabetics. People who have this syndrome are usually overweight, have hyperinsulinaemia and insulin resistance, high cholesterol and/or high triglyceride levels, as well as high blood pressure
◆ Possible development of insulin resistance in otherwise healthy people
◆ Possible polycystic ovaries in women, with concomitant low fertility and hyperlipidemia (high cholesterol and/or high triglyceride levels)
◆ Continuous hunger pangs, resulting from blood glucose levels "screaming up one side of the witch's hat and crashing down the other side" – the so-called blood glucose roller coaster (see page 81 for explanation)
◆ Possible exacerbation of candida infections in those prone to it
◆ Increased blood pressure, in the long term
◆ Longstanding overweight, which seems to be resistant to efforts at weight loss.

2. Helps to prevent diabetes and the micro- and macro-vascular damage caused by poor blood glucose control

As explained before, eating high-GI foods all the time can predispose to diabetes. High blood glucose levels, per se, are also very damaging to the body. In nature, all reducing sugars (sugars that consist of one molecule, such as glucose, fructose and galactose) have an affinity for, and will readily bind with, available proteins. This happens, for example, when a cake is baked. The sugars in the batter bind with the proteins (milk and egg) in the batter and give the cake the appetising brown surface we associate with the cake being ready.

Likewise, in the body, when blood glucose levels are above 8,5 mmol/l, the glucose (a reducing sugar) will tend to bind with body proteins. This process is called *glycosylation*. Once glucose is bound to a body protein, it hampers the protein from functioning normally, and if many body proteins are affected in this way, some body systems will start to malfunction.

The proteins in the lens of the eye, for example, will bind with free glucose if blood glucose levels are high for any period of time. This results in the lens becoming opaque, a condition known as cataracts. This is the reason so many uncontrolled diabetics develop eye and vision problems. In the same way, glucose can also bind to the proteins in the walls of the cells lining our blood vessels, thereby decreasing cell wall flexibility, which is one of the first steps in the development of cardiovascular disease. In addition, high blood glucose levels raise triglyceride levels, another risk factor for heart disease.

So it becomes obvious that we need to be aware that our blood glucose or fuel levels play a vital role in our wellbeing, both in the short and long term.

3. Improved weight loss

When we abuse our body's ability to regulate blood glucose levels, our bodies will eventually "burn out" and no longer be able to regulate blood glucose levels properly.

Overweight and obesity are often caused by incorrect eating, in terms of both the *type* and the *quantity* of food eaten. How often have you heard someone lament: "But I really eat like a bird. I just have to *look* at food and put on weight!" Although this isn't literally true, some people do have a real physiological problem, continuing to put on weight even though they may be eating very little. Let us explain.

When we eat a high-GI food such as toast, rice cakes, cornflakes, potatoes, bread rolls, etc., our blood glucose level will rise sharply within the next 30 to 60 minutes. The body likes to function within a very narrow range of blood glucose levels, and when the level is exceeded, it will do everything it can to get back to the ideal level (4 – 7.8 mmol/l).

In the case of high blood glucose levels, the body responds by sending a signal to the pancreas to produce insulin to clear the excess glucose from the blood, into the body cells. If this sharp rise in blood glucose is repeated often enough, the pancreas will eventually over-produce insulin in response to the stimulation it receives as a result of the high glucose levels.

The pancreas becomes frantic, trying to keep up with the continuous surges of excess glucose. In its hurry to produce enough insulin, the pancreas sends out the insulin before it's properly formed, and we end up with excess "incomplete" insulin in the bloodstream; the "incomplete" insulin is unable to transport the blood glucose to the cells.

The body then responds by making more insulin, driving the beta cells in the pancreas to near exhaustion. More "incomplete" insulin is produced in response to the still-high blood glucose levels and we end up with continuous high insulin levels (hyperinsulinaemia) with concomitant insulin resistance.

Insulin stores fat, so if huge quantities of insulin are secreted day after day by your pancreas, it's not surprising that you will put on weight or have difficulty losing weight.

So what is the key to controlling and preventing hyperinsulinaemia and insulin resistance, and all the consequences? Treat the root cause, i.e. control your blood glucose level and watch your fat intake!

The type of carbohydrate you eat can affect your blood glucose level and, therefore, how much insulin your body has to produce. So to keep insulin levels within normal metabolic parameters and thereby control your weight, it's imperative that you select mainly those carbohydrates that give an even blood glucose response – foods low on the Glycemic Index – and keep your fat intake in check (because fat causes insulin to work less effectively).

In practice, the obvious answer to getting out of this vicious fat-storing cycle is to break free and eat only low-GI, lower-fat foods at every meal, until the pancreas realises it no longer needs to produce huge quantities of insulin to control blood glucose levels. This will reduce the high levels of insulin in the blood and the accompanying insulin resistance, which will result in weight loss.

Eating low-GI meals thus has a marked impact on the body's ability to lose weight.

If we eat low-GI, lower-fat meals:

◆ There's no marked rise in blood glucose levels,
◆ no excess insulin production,
◆ no lipoprotein lipase (LPL)
  and therefore
◆ no fat storage.

In addition, because low-GI foods are absorbed so much slower, they're very filling and satisfying and you retain a sense of fullness for at least three hours. Combine this with a little protein and fat (see "Putting it all together", page 116), and you won't get hungry for five to six hours after you've eaten. This will stop you feeling hungry between meals, and you automatically eat less.

Consider the opposite of this. When you eat a high-GI meal, your blood glucose level rises dramatically and then falls again, just as dramatically, to below your starting blood glucose level (see graph on page 81). The result of this dramatic fall in blood glucose level is that you get very hungry. The natural response would be to eat, so you grab a pie or a doughnut (high GI, high fat) and send your blood glucose level soaring again. Not only have you eaten between meals, adding extra fat and energy to your daily intake, but you've also chosen a high-fat food which is immediately stored as a result of the release of large quantities of insulin in response to the glucose surge.

And if these two reasons don't convince you, then consider that most low-GI foods take longer to eat and give your satiety signal time to kick in, which means you will automatically eat less, because you'll feel full long before you can overeat. Low-GI portions are thus self-limiting, and for this reason we don't encourage you to weigh your food. Besides, it's far too tedious to have to weigh everything you eat. (See page 117 for portion control made easy.)

A good example is a lunch made up of two slices of ordinary brown bread, spread with low-fat mayonnaise, and topped with ham and tomato to make a single, high-fat, high-GI sandwich. This can be wolfed down in a minute, assuming you are very hungry. Replace the high-GI bread with slices of a dense, firm loaf of bread such as seed loaf and you'll have trouble finishing the second slice of bread. See what we mean by self-limiting?

So, there are many very good reasons why it's important to learn about the Glycemic Index in order to lose weight successfully:

- ◆ Low-GI meals ensure small, but steady blood glucose release
- ◆ Low-GI meals don't over-stimulate insulin secretion
- ◆ Low-GI meals keep the secretion of lipoprotein lipase (LPL) in check
- ◆ Low-GI meals keep you feeling full for much longer
- ◆ Low-GI meals stop you getting hungry between meals
- ◆ Low-GI meals stop you eating unnecessary snacks between meals
- ◆ Low-GI meals help you eat less at every meal.

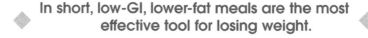

In short, low-GI, lower-fat meals are the most effective tool for losing weight.

4. Enhancement of sports performance:

(See also Sport nutrition guidelines [page 179])

Excellence at sport is all about optimising your energy reserves and sources during training, events and (especially) after sports to minimise exhaustion, increase endurance and speed up recovery. This applies equally to the serious, and the more casual, sportsman and woman, such as those who regularly go for a brisk walk, or attend an aerobics session most days of the week. Exercise is such an integral part of a weight loss and healthy living programme, that it's worth your while to pay attention to this next section.

Maximising enjoyment and performance in sport or an exercise programme simply means choosing the form of exercise that's right for you, and optimising your blood glucose control. This task is made relatively easy with the help of the Glycemic Index information we have on hand.

During exercise you need a good, steady supply of fuel (energy) so that your muscles can keep working at peak performance. Remember that the fuel source for your body is glucose, which comes mainly from carbohydrates, so it makes sense to eat low GI, or slow-release carbohydrates, before exercise so that you have a steady stream of glucose available throughout the exercise session or event.

Examples of suitable low GI pre-exercise meals include:
◆ Fruit salad with low-fat or fat-free yoghurt
◆ A low GI cereal with low-fat or fat-free milk
◆ Baked beans on toast with a little grated low-fat cheese, if desired
◆ Fettucine napoleatana (pasta with low-fat herb and tomato sauce).

For more low-GI foods and meals, see meals for one week starting on page 156, the GI lists starting on page 213, the recipes starting on on page 191, and the lower-GI recipe book *Eating for Sustained Energy* by Liesbet Delport and Gabi Steenkamp.

Eating a low-GI meal or snack before exercising means that the body has a steady supply of glucose for up to three hours after eating. Many people think that drinking a high-GI sports drink before an event will help with their performance; in fact, the opposite is true! Blood glucose levels shoot up, but within 30 minutes they come crashing down to leave you without any fuel (energy) half an hour into your event. Not really what you're looking for! (The graph on page 93 shows what happens to blood glucose levels if you drink a high-GI sports drink before exercise.)

To top up your energy supply during a longer bout of exercise (lasting longer than 90 minutes), your body will need an immediate source of fuel, and this is readily available from intermediate or high GI carbohydrates. As it's difficult to eat during exercise, drinking an intermediate- or high-GI drink – such as cordials, fruit juices, soft drinks, sports drinks, etc. – is the practical solution.

The most critical aspect of applying this GI information is *what you eat or drink* within 10 – 30 minutes after finishing the exercise. Your muscle glycogen stores will be depleted, and your muscles will "suck" as much glucose from your blood as they can to replenish it.

This is also called the "sponge effect", because of the working of the enzyme, glycogen resynthetase, after exercise. The result is a very rapid drop in blood glucose levels, which needs to be replenished to avoid fatigue and exhaustion. That shaky feeling, those wobbly legs or the desire to sleep after exercise are signs of your blood glucose level plummeting.

High-GI drinks and foods are ideal for topping up glycogen stores after exercise. Some examples include:

◆ Chilled, sliced melon or a bowl of melon balls
◆ A bowl of tropical fruit salad made up of melons, papino and pineapple, finely diced and chilled
◆ A high-GI cereal (for example, Weetbix, chocolate Pronutro) and low-fat or fat-free milk with sugar, if desired
◆ Any one of the high-GI energy drinks or fruit juices on the market.

When GIFSA tested the effects of a high-GI sports drink on the blood glucose level of a healthy person after exercise, the blood glucose response was the same as if a low-GI drink had been consumed. See the graphs below, which compare the effect of a high-GI drink on someone who hasn't exercised, and the effect of the same drink, on the same person, after exercise.

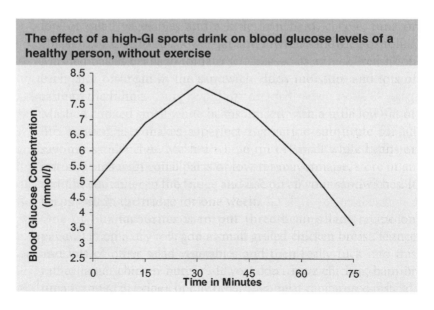

The effect of a high-GI sports drink on blood glucose levels of a healthy person, without exercise

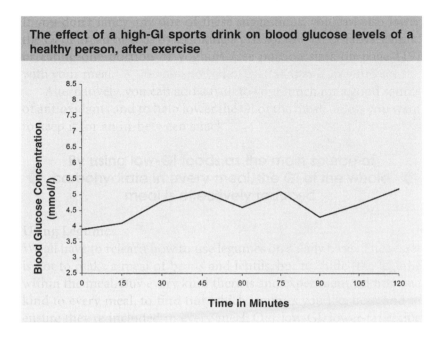

The effect of a high-GI sports drink on blood glucose levels of a healthy person, after exercise

After looking at these graphs, it also becomes obvious why exercise is so important in controlling blood glucose levels in those suffering from insulin resistance, hypoglycaemia, hyperinsulinaemia and diabetes. There is one proviso: diabetics should stick to intermediate-GI foods and drinks to replenish muscle glycogen stores after exercise, as their insulin is not as efficient in placing the glucose in cells, unless they were active for two hours or more.

5. Other advantages or benefits

Eating the low-GI, lower-fat way helps to:
- Lower cholesterol levels
- Lower triglyceride levels
- Reduce high blood pressure
- Ameliorate ADHD (attention deficit hyperactivity disorder). Consult a dietician for the other factors that have to be kept in mind for this condition.
- Prevent and treat polycystic ovarian syndrome (PCOS)
- Treat chronic candida infections. Candida is a yeast that thrives on high blood sugar levels, not sugar per se, in the gastrointestinal

tract, so it's not necessary to exclude sugar from the diet. By simply following a low-GI diet, blood glucose levels are kept at normal levels and candida can no longer thrive. Consult a dietician for other factors that have to be considered.

Chapter 5

Fat

Fat intake questionnaire

How slim and trim is your daily intake?

Answer the questions below, relating to what you normally eat in a typical week. Circle the answer that best suits your situation. Check your score for each answer at the end of the questionnaire and add up your scores. Your total score will give you an indication of how successfully (or unsuccessfully) you're fat-proofing your diet.

It's quite an interesting exercise to repeat this questionnaire after you've followed the eating plan for a month, and see by how much you've improved your score.

1. In a typical week, how many milkshakes, iced coffees, Dom Pedros, Irish coffees and standard ice creams do you consume?

a. None
b. 1
c. 2
d. 3
e. 4 or more

2. In a typical week, how many pieces of cake, muffins, rusks and biscuits do you eat?

Count two to three plain biscuits, such as Marie biscuits, as one unit, and one double biscuit, such as Romany Creams, or a rich biscuit, such as shortbread, as one unit.

a. None
b. 1 per week
c. 2 per week
d. 3 per week
e. 4 per week
f. 5 or more per week

3. In a typical week, how many chocolate bars, chocolate slabs and squares of fudge do you eat? Count one for every small chocolate bar, one third of a 100 g slab of chocolate and every 4 cm square of fudge.

a. None
b. 1
c. 2
d. 3
e. More than 3

4. In a typical week, how many small packets of crisps (30 g) do you eat?

a. None
b. 1
c. 2
d. 3
e. More than 3

5. In a typical week, how many handfuls of nuts and/or seeds do you eat? (Peanuts, Brazil nuts, cashew nuts, etc., pumpkin seeds, sunflower seeds, etc.)

a. None
b. 1
c. 2
d. 3
e. 4 or more

6. In a typical week, how many times do you have hot chips, including those made at home, eaten in restaurants or bought as take-aways (deep-fried, potato wedges or oven-baked)?

a. Never
b. Once
c. Twice
d. 3 or more times
e. 4 or more times

7. In a typical week, how many take-away meals do you have? (Pies, pastries, deep-fried chicken, toasted sandwiches, schwarmas, hamburgers and pizzas)

a. None
b. 1
c. 2
d. 3
e. 4
f. 5 or more

8. In a typical week, how many salads do you eat with standard dressing, low-fat dressing or olive oil? You may wish to circle more than one answer.

a. 1 with a standard dressing and/or olive oil
b. 1 with a low-fat dressing
c. 2 with a standard dressing and/or olive oil
d. 2 with a low-fat dressing
e. 3 with a standard dressing and/or olive oil
f. 3 with a low-fat dressing
g. None
h. More than 3 with standard dressing and/or olive oil
i. More than 3 with low-fat dressing

9. How many times a week do you eat red meat? (Beef, mutton, lamb, pork; for example steak, chops, roasts, bacon, stews, casseroles)

a. Never
b. 5 or more times
c. 3 to 4 times
d. Twice
e. Once

10. In a typical week, how often do you use cream? (In or on a pudding or dessert, in soups, casseroles, Irish coffees, on a potato, with scones or muffins, in a cappuccino, in a choccacino, etc.; at dinner parties)

a. Never
b. Once
c. Twice
d. 3 times
e. 4 times
f. 5 or more times

11. Think about the last two days: how many teaspoons of butter and/or margarine and/or peanut butter and/or oil did you use (for frying, spreading on bread and toast, baking, spreading on scones and/or muffins, toasting sandwiches, etc.)? If you used peanut butter or lite margarine, count 2 teaspoons as one.

a. None
b. 1 – 2 tsp
c. 2 – 4 tsp
d. 4 – 6 tsp
e. 6 – 8 tsp
f. 8 or more teaspoons

12. How often do you eat avocado?

a. Never
b. Occasionally
c. Once a month
d. 2 – 3 times a month
e. Once a week
f. 2 – 3 times a week
g. Every day
h. Twice a day

13. How often do you eat an English breakfast (eggs and bacon)?

a. Never
b. Occasionally
c. 2 – 3 times a month
d. Once a week
e. Twice a week
f. 3 or more times a week

14. Which statement is most applicable to you?

a. I usually remove the fat on meat and the skin of chicken *before* cooking.
b. I usually remove the fat on meat or the skin of chicken (not both) *before* cooking.
c. I usually remove the fat on meat and/or the skin of chicken *after* cooking.
d. I never remove the fat on meat or the skin of chicken.

15. How many times a week do you eat puddings or other desserts?

a. Never
b. Once
c. Twice
d. 3 times
e. 4 or more times

16. Do you generally use standard mayonnaise or lite/lower-fat mayonnaise?

a. Standard mayonnaise
b. Lite or lower-fat mayonnaise
c. Both
d. None

17. How often do you eat out? (In restaurants or at friends' dinner parties)

a. Never
b. Occasionally
c. Once a month
d. Two or three times a month
e. Once a week
f. Twice a week
g. More than twice a week

18. When eating out in restaurants, do you ...

a. Order a main course only
b. Order a starter and a main course
c. Order a main course and a dessert
d. Order a starter, a main course and a dessert
e. Order a starter only
f. Order a pudding only
g. Order 2 starters (1 as a main meal)
h. Don't eat out in restaurants

19. When you eat out, what do you usually order? You may need to circle more than one answer.

a. Spare ribs, boerewors, lamb/mutton, fried chops, grilled chicken, oxtail, snails in garlic butter, seafood cocktail, creamy soup
b. Grilled ladies' steak (even for a man), grilled fish or calamari, chicken or beef kebabs, Parma ham
c. Crumbed or deep-fried foods (e.g. mushrooms, calamari, schnitzel, etc.)
d. Chips, fried rice, potato wedges
e. Rice, baked potato or pasta
f. None of the above

20. As a rule, do you use ...

a. Full-cream milk
b. 2% or low-fat milk
c. Skimmed milk
d. Low-fat milk and skimmed milk
e. No milk

21. As a rule, what kinds of cheeses do you eat?

a. Standard/full-cream cheeses
b. Medium-fat cheeses e.g. mozzarella, feta, In Shape
c. Lower-fat cheeses (<12% fat) e.g. Lichten Blanc, cottage cheese (not cream cheese)
d. No cheese
e. Lower-fat and standard cheeses

22. What kind of yoghurt do you generally eat?

a. Double cream (fruit or plain)
b. Full-cream (fruit or plain)
c. Low-fat 2% (fruit or plain)
d. Fat-free (fruit or plain)
e. Don't eat yoghurt

23. Do you know how to "fake-fry"?
(i.e. fry food in only one drop of oil)

a. Yes
b. No

24. Circle the appropriate statements about cottage cheese and cream cheese below. You may wish to circle more than one answer.

a. Cream cheese, cottage cheese, and creamed cottage cheese all have the same fat content
b. Cottage cheese contains much less fat than cream cheese
c. I eat mainly cottage cheese
d. I eat mainly cream cheese
e. I don't eat cottage cheese or cream cheese.

25. How many times a week do you eat processed meats, such as Vienna sausages, polony, salami, pepperoni, Russians, frankfurters, käsegriller, German franks, bacon, etc.? You can halve your score if you eat the lower-fat version.

a. Never
b. Once a week
c. Twice a week
d. 3 – 4 times a week
e. Every day

26. How often do you eat toasted muesli? (Not combined with another cereal)

a. Never
b. Once a week
c. Once or twice a week
d. 3 times a week
e. Every day, or more than 3 times a week

27. How often do you have sauces with your meals in a typical week?

a. Never
b. 1 – 2 times a week
c. 3 – 4 times a week
d. 5+ times a week

28. How many meals per week contain hard cheese (Cheddar, Gouda, Edam, etc.)?

a. None
b. 1 a week
c. 2 a week
d. 3 – 5 a week
e. 5+ a week

29. How often do you eat dried wors and biltong?

a. Never, or occasionally
b. Only lean biltong
c. Once a week (wors/biltong)
d. More than 3 times a week

30. How often do you eat deep-fat fried foods? (Schnitzel, chicken nuggets, deep-fried fish, deep-fried onion rings, deep-fried mushrooms, deep-fried calamari, etc.)

a. Never, or occasionally
b. Once or twice a week
c. 3 times a week
d. 5 or more times a week

Scoring

1. Milkshakes, iced coffee and ice cream
    a. 0
    b. 1
    c. 2
    d. 3
    e. 5

2. Cake, muffins and biscuits
    a. 0
    b. 1
    c. 2
    d. 3
    e. 4
    f. 5

3. Chocolate and fudge
    a. 0
    b. 2
    c. 4
    d. 6
    e. 8

4. Crisps
    a. 0
    b. 2
    c. 4
    d. 6
    e. 8

5. Nuts and seeds
    a. 0
    b. 1
    c. 2
    d. 3
    e. 4

6. Hot chips
    a. 0
    b. 1
    c. 2
    d. 3
    e. 5

7. Pies and pastries
    a. 0
    b. 1
    c. 2
    d. 3
    e. 4
    f. 5

8. Salad dressing
    a. 1
    b. 0
    c. 2
    d. 1
    e. 3
    f. 2
    g. 0
    h. 5
    i. 3

9. Red meat
   a. 0
   b. 6
   c. 3
   d. 2
   e. 1

10. Cream
   a. 0
   b. 1
   c. 2
   d. 3
   e. 4
   f. 5

11. Butter and margarine
   a. 0
   b. 1
   c. 2
   d. 3
   e. 4
   f. 6

12. Avocado
   a. 0
   b. 0
   c. 1
   d. 2
   e. 3
   f. 4
   g. 5
   h. 6

13. Egg and bacon
   a. 0
   b. 1
   c. 2
   d. 3
   e. 4
   f. 5

14. Removing visible fat
   a. 0
   b. 2
   c. 3
   d. 4

15. Dessert/pudding
   a. 0
   b. 1
   c. 2
   d. 3
   e. 5

16. Mayonnaise
   a. 4
   b. 2
   c. 3
   d. 0

17. Eating out
   a. 0
   b. 1
   c. 2
   d. 3
   e. 4
   f. 6
   g. 8

18. Restaurant choices
    a. 3
    b. 4
    c. 4
    d. 5
    e. 2
    f. 3
    g. 4
    h. 0

19. Restaurant orders
    a. 5
    b. 3
    c. 5
    d. 5
    e. 2
    f. 2

20. Milk
    a. 4
    b. 2
    c. 0
    d. 1
    e. 0

21. Cheeses
    a. 4
    b. 2
    c. 1
    d. 0
    e. 3

22. Yoghurt
    a. 5
    b. 4
    c. 1
    d. 0
    e. 0

23. Fake-frying
    a. 0
    b. 2

24. Cottage and cream cheese
    a. 2
    b. 0
    c. 1
    d. 3
    e. 0

25. Processed meats
    a. 0
    b. 1
    c. 2
    d. 3
    e. 5

26. Toasted muesli
    a. 0
    b. 1
    c. 2
    d. 3
    e. 5

27. Sauces
    a. 0
    b. 1
    c. 4
    d. 5

29. Biltong
    a. 0
    b. 1
    c. 2
    d. 6

28. Hard cheeses
    a. 0
    b. 1
    c. 2
    d. 4
    e. 5

30. Deep-fat fried foods
    a. 0
    b. 2
    c. 4
    d. 6

Now add up your scores for each answer to get a total score. Read on to find out how well you are fat-proofing your diet.

Totals

Below 25

Your fat intake is too low. Research has shown that the human body needs fat to function properly and to lose weight. Too low fat intakes are detrimental to your health. Make sure you familiarise yourself with the lower-fat choices and use them instead of the no-fat or fat-free choices you've been used to in the past.

Below 40

Well done; this score means you're making good lower-fat choices and controlling your intake to the correct degree for weight loss. Keep it up! If you're female, your score should preferably be around 40, and if you're male, up to 50 is fine. If you want to maintain your weight and your score falls into this category, your fat intake might be slightly too low, so don't cut down any further.

40 – 60

This score indicates a medium fat intake, which shows you're making an effort in our modern take-away society. But you need to work a little harder at familiarising yourself with the lower-fat choices you can make, and then put this into practice. If you want to lose weight, you'll have to lower your fat intake effectively, so your food choices definitely need attention. This score is fine for weight maintenance, where women should fall between 40 and 50, and men between 50 and 60.

60+

Wow – what can we say? Your fat intake is *far* too high and you need to learn all about making better lower-fat choices. Read the entire section on fat carefully, as well as the sections on fat-proofing your diet (page 132), label-reading skills (page 141) and eating out (page 151). Make sure you absorb this information and put it into practice every day.

You'll be amazed at how easy this can be – all the tips given in this book are simple and easy to follow. Good luck!

Now that you know where you stand at present, read on to find out how to improve your nutritional intake, be healthier and lose the weight you've been wanting to lose for so long.

Why do you need to follow a lower-fat diet?

◆ Fat is fattening! During the 1980s, a group of researchers conducted a study in which various sources of fat were fed to different subjects, i.e. some ate nuts, others avocado, others chocolates, etc. When biopsies were taken of the body fat, it was found that the body fat of those who ate the nuts had almost the same structure as the fat of the nuts, the body fat of those who ate avocado resembled the fat of avocado, and those who ate chocolate had a body fat composition similar to chocolate fat, etc. From this we can learn two things:

1. It doesn't require much effort for the body to convert dietary fat into body fat.
   i.e. *Fat makes us fat!*
2. The body makes use of all fat ingested, even if it is "bad" or unhealthy fat, and this, in turn, predisposes us to all sorts of degenerative diseases, e.g. cancer, heart disease, arthritis, etc.

◆ In addition, *a high-fat diet in itself inevitably predisposes us to lifestyle diseases* such as overweight, diabetes, high blood pressure, high blood lipid levels, hyperinsulinaemia, insulin resistance, polycystic ovarian syndrome, gout and cancer.

One recent meta-analysis of lower-fat diets concluded that a reduction of 10% in the proportion of energy from fat (without any other changes in diet or lifestyle) was associated with a reduction in weight of 16 g a day, corresponding to a reduction of 1,4 kg in body weight over three months, or 2,8 kg over 6 months. This may seem like a small weight loss, but compared to the gradual increase in body weight many people experience over time (if you pick up 1 kg weight a month, you pick up 12 kg per year!), a weight loss of even a few kilograms is important, especially when there is no kilojoule (energy) restriction involved in achieving this weight loss. If you watch your portions (especially fat portions) and your total food intake, and increase activity, you will lose more weight.

See the section on label-reading skills for tips on watching out for the fat content of foods (page 141).

Sorting out beneficial and detrimental fats

As explained in the section on fad diets, we cannot exclude all fats from our daily diet. All healthy diets must contain adequate quantities of essential fatty acids, since these are fats our bodies cannot make. These essential fatty acids include both Omega-3 and Omega-6, which are both polyunsaturated fatty acids (PUFAs). They are very important, as they are the building blocks of important hormones that regulate essential biological functions.

Usually you'll get plenty of **Omega-6 fatty acids** (of which linoleic acid is the most important) from low-fat protein sources such as tuna and chicken, vegetable oils such as sunflower oil, soft margarine in tubs, low-oil mayonnaise/salad dressing, whole-grain products and a few seeds and nuts. Omega-6 PUFAs help prevent and cure water retention, eczema, attention deficit hyperactivity disorder (ADHD) and high blood cholesterol levels.

Unless you eat a lot of cold water fish (fatty fish such as pilchards and salmon), linseeds and linseed (flax) oil or canola oil, you probably won't take in enough **Omega-3 fatty acids** (of which linolenic acid is the most important). Omega-3 PUFAs can help prevent and alleviate thrombosis, ADHD, high blood pressure, gout and arthritis. They also have a beneficial effect on general heart health and may even help to control insulin levels.

Monosaturated fatty acids (MUFAs) are also important. These fats have been shown to lower both total cholesterol and triglyceride levels without lowering the levels of "good" HDL cholesterol, which improves cardiac risk profiles more effectively than some fat-free diets. Olive oil and palm oil (called "Carotino" oil in South Africa) contain appreciable quantities of natural antioxidants. Monosaturated fats such as olive oil, canola oil, almonds, peanuts, avocado pears and olives also play a critical role in controlling insulin secretion, because they slow the rate at which carbohydrates are digested and enter your blood stream. Ironically, this enables you to tap into your stored body fat for energy more effectively – remember, it takes some fat to burn fat!

So, contrary to what we've been told over the past few years, healthy fat in your diet is very important to your health and aids in fat loss. Healthy fats should be incorporated into every meal, every day. Just keep in mind that all fats, even healthy fats, are fattening and that is why the energy from fat shouldn't be more than 30% of your total daily energy intake.

The most harmful fat is **saturated fat**. Unfortunately, saturated fats are also those most commonly consumed in excess. The fat on meat, the skin on chicken, deep-fried food, butter, lard, cream, cheese, full-cream milk, full-cream yoghurt, ice cream, crisps, Brazil nuts, coconut, brick margarine, coffee and tea creamers and anything containing coconut oil and palm kernel oil, are all sources of saturated fats. (Note that palm oil is a "good" fat and palm kernel oil a "bad" fat.) A few plant foods are sources of saturated fats, as mentioned above: Brazil nuts, brick margarine, coffee and tea creamers, coconut, coconut oil and palm kernel oil. The body uses these fats to make the "bad" LDL cholesterol, which blocks arteries. They also play a role in cancer and arthritis.

Other "new" detrimental fats are **trans-fatty acids**, which are formed when *any* kind of fat is repeatedly heated. Heat causes a change in the structure of the fatty acids, which renders them inactive and useless to the body. Not only are trans-fatty acids of no use to the body, but they can also interfere with many metabolic processes, do damage in our bodies and make us more prone to any of the lifestyle diseases, such as cancer, heart disease, suppressed immunity, etc. The most common sources of these detrimental trans-fatty acids are deep-fat fried foods such as hot chips, deep-fried onion rings, fried crumbed fish, fried chicken pieces, fried calamari, etc. prepared in fast-food outlets and restaurants. So now you have two very good reasons to avoid fried foods when eating out – the high fat content as well as the trans-fatty acids!

How much fat is healthy?

If you stick to our guidelines and add only one fat per meal, you will easily keep to the following recommended quantities of total fat, as well as to the good types of fat. If you want to maintain your weight, you can consume a little bit more fat, as explained in the scoring section of the fat intake questionnaire (page 106).

See Label-reading skills (page 141) to learn how to keep within these recommendations, even if you have to prepare meals in a hurry, using many ready-prepared products. Please note that these recommended quantities can vary with individual needs, so it is best to see a dietician who will be able to tell you exactly how much you need every day. See GIFSA's website (www.gifoundation.com) for a list of dieticians who use the Glycemic Index in their treatment.

Recommended quantities of the different types of fat

As a general guide, you should make sure that most of the fat you eat is **mono-unsaturated** (canola or olive oil, peanuts, almonds, pecans, macadamias, cashews, peanut butter, olives and avocado). This type of fat should make up at least 30% of your total fat intake, or 10% of your total kilojoule intake.

Try, also, to consume good sources of Omega-3 **polyunsaturated fats** ("fatty" fish such as pilchards, trout, etc., linseed and canola oil) on a regular basis. If you don't eat at least two to three servings a week of fatty fish such as pilchards, sardines, trout, galjoen or yellowtail, or use linseed oil (flax oil) in your food, you can take fish oil or Omega-3 supplements, as Omega-3 fatty acids may help control insulin levels and protect against inflammatory disease such as arthritis. If in doubt, consult your dietitian

Supplemental fish oil (salmon oil is rich in Omega-3 fatty acids) can be taken in amounts up to 3 g (3 000 mg) a day. It's also a good idea to supplement with natural vitamin E, which helps the Omega-3 fatty acids to work even better. Based on the most recent research, we recommend you take 100 to 200 IU (international units) of natural vitamin E every day. It's important to check that the vitamin E you take is d-alpha tocopherol, the technical name for natural vitamin E, as this is the only form in which the body can use vitamin E efficiently.

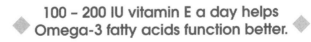

**100 – 200 IU vitamin E a day helps
Omega-3 fatty acids function better.**

Try to limit the use of the **Omega-6 polyunsaturated fats**, found in most vegetable oils and tub margarines, as the typical western diet contains about 10 times more Omega-6 than Omega-3 fatty acids, while the ideal ratio is thought to be 2 – 4:1 (and not 10:1). The total quantity of polyunsaturated fats, including both Omega-3 and Omega-6, should also make up about 30% of your total fat intake, or

10% of your total kilojoule intake. Try, however, to concentrate more on consuming Omega-3 fatty acids.

Try not to use **saturated fats** (butter, lard, cream, brick margarine, coconut milk/cream, etc.), and sources of trans-fatty acids, such as deep-fat fried foods. To help you accomplish this, limit red meat intake to a maximum of three times a week. Most of our clients find it helpful to allocate three specific days of the week to red meat. Even when they're eating out, they stick to the "red meat day" rule, and choose red meat dishes from the menu only if it is a red meat day. If they're invited out on a non-red meat day, they simply choose fish or chicken from the menu. If you don't like this idea, or find it impossible to stick to, you'll have to compensate; for example, if you have red meat on a fish or chicken day, you'll have to have fish or chicken on one of your red meat days.

Recommended quantities of total fat

Internationally, low-fat foods are defined as those containing 3 g fat or less per 100 g of food, and fat-free foods are those that contain 0,5 g fat or less per 100 g food.

Many dieticians, all over the world, advise their clients to give preference to foods that contain 10 g fat per 100 g of food, as it is very difficult to stick to the international recommendation of eating only low-fat foods (those that contain 3% fat or less).

The practical fat intake – which boils down to eating smart and staying slim – lies somewhere between 3% and 10%. This is what we call lower-fat eating. It's more realistic and is a recommendation that you will easily be able to follow for the rest of your life.

As a rule, we recommend that you try to keep to about *10 g to 13 g of fat per meal. Women should definitely keep to this recommendation and men should not consume more than 17 g fat per meal.*

In practical terms this means that you may only have *one* added fat in any one meal, which leaves a little spare for the fat contained in the protein. Your starch and vegetables should preferably not contain any fat.

The general health recommendation is:

◆ 30 g – 50 g of fat a day for those wishing to lose weight
(30 g – 40 g fat for women, and 40 g – 50 g for men)

◆ 40 g – 60 g fat for those on a weight maintenance plan
(40 g – 50 g for women, and 50 g – 60 g for men).

Considering saturated fats only, one third of this translates into about *10 g – 13 g* saturated fats a day for *women*, and *13 g – 17 g* saturated fats a day for *men*.

The table below shows the fat content of some common foods, in the portion sizes normally eaten. An *asterisk (*)* next to a food means that it is a *high-fat food*, and should thus only be consumed on special occasions. *Two asterisks (**)* mean the food is *very high in fat*, and should preferably be avoided altogether, or eaten only on very special occasions – say, once a year!

Fat content of some typical protein foods

Please note that the fat content of foods is given for typical food portion sizes

Food	Serving size	Grams of fat per serving
Beef fillet, grilled, fat trimmed	120 g (palm of hand)	11,2 g
Beef fillet, grilled, not trimmed**	120 g	20,6 g**
Beef fillet, grilled, fat trimmed	150 g (ladies' steak)	14,0 g
Beef fillet, grilled, not trimmed**	150 g (ladies' steak)	25,8 g**
Rump steak, fried, fat trimmed	120 g (palm of hand)	10,3 g
Rump steak, fried, not trimmed**	120 g	20,5 g**
Rump steak, grilled, fat trimmed	150 g (ladies' steak)	9,3 g
Rump steak, grilled, not trimmed**	150 g (ladies' steak)	25,6 g**
Mince, standard*	100 g (3 heaped T)	18,9 g*
Mince, lean (topside will be less)	100 g (3 heaped T)	11,3 g
Boerewors (beef sausage)**	100 g (10 cm piece)	36,3 g**
Traditional pork sausage**	75 g (1 sausage)	23,4 g**
Pork banger (15% fat)	55 g (1 sausage)	9,4 g
Pork chop, grilled, fat trimmed	100 g (1 loin chop)	15,3 g
Pork roast, not trimmed**	100 g (3 thin slices)	20,7 g**
Spare ribs (pork)**	120 g (6 ribs)	36,4 g**
Kassler rib chops, grilled, fat trimmed	100 g (palm of hand)	8,4 g

Mutton chop, grilled, not trimmed**	120 g (palm of hand)	27,7 g**
Mutton, roasted, fat trimmed*	100 g (3 thin slices)	16,5 g*
Chicken breast, roasted, with skin*	150 g (1 average breast)	16,4 g*
Chicken breast, roasted, no skin	150 g (1 average breast)	6,8 g
Chicken thigh, roasted, with skin*	100 g (1 thigh)	15,8 g*
Chicken thigh, roasted, no skin	100 g (1 thigh)	9,7 g
Deep-fried chicken**	150 g (1 breast)	26,1 g**
Deep-fried chicken*	100 g (1 thigh)	17,4 g*
Deep-fried chicken*	108 g (6 nuggets)	17,5 g*
Turkey, roasted, with skin	100 g (3 thin slices)	9,7 g
Egg, boiled	60 g (1 large)	6,2 g
Ham, lean	50 g (2 slices)	2,5 g
Vienna sausage	40 g (1 Vienna)	10,1 g
Lean Vienna sausage	40 g (1 Vienna)	3,5 g
Polony	50 g (2 slices)	14,13 g
Salami*	50 g (5 thin slices)	17,25 g*
Bacon, lean, fat removed	40 g (3 cooked rashers)	9,0 g
Bacon, streaky, fried*	40 g (3 fried rashers)	19,6 g*

When you look at this table closely, you will see that rump steak, grilled (fat trimmed), is leaner than the same quantity of fillet steak; this is true even for a larger portion. If, however, you eat rump or fillet steak *with* the fat, the difference in fat content between the two is negligible. Boerewors and pork spare ribs are higher in fat than deep-fat fried chicken, and a deep-fat fried chicken thigh contains less fat than a deep-fat fried chicken breast. All of these are far too high in fat to be eaten regularly, however; we're merely pointing out that we must all become very fat conscious and not just believe what we're told.

You can also see, quite clearly, from the table that red meat is high in fat, particularly saturated or "bad" fats. For this reason we recommend that red meat be eaten no more than three times a week, in small portions. If you stick to this, it will be easy to keep the fat content of each meal within the recommended limit (not more than 10 g – 13 g fat per meal for women and not more than 13 g – 17 g fat per meal for men). Including red meat in any meal (even lean and grilled) automatically brings the fat content of that meal to the recommended level. This means that you should not add any fat to meals containing red meat. If, however, you didn't have any fat at one of your meals earlier that day – breakfast, for example – you could still add *one* good-quality fat to the meal containing red meat. Men might still be able to add an extra "good" fat, but not if they eat a "male portion" of red meat in a restaurant.

To help you keep within the fat recommendations, see the section on fat-proofing your meals (page 132). You will also benefit from a consultation with a dietician, who will help you determine exactly how to trim the fat within your healthy lifestyle.

What about cheese?

Most full-cream cheeses contain about 30% fat. This means they have 30 g of fat per 100 g portion. In reality, most people only eat 30 g – one matchbox full – on a slice of bread or on a roll. This is why 30 g of cheese is generally regarded as one portion. Let's take a look at some common cheeses and their fat content per "matchbox" of cheese (30 g).

Fat content of some typical cheeses	
Cheese	**Grams fat per 30 g cheese** One "matchbox" of cheese
Lower-fat cheese	
Cottage cheese, fat-free	0,15 – 0,3 g
Cottage cheese, low-fat (3 T)	1,5 g
Creamed cottage cheese	3,0 g
Medium-fat cottage cheese	3,0 g
Processed cheese wedges (2)	3,0 g
Cheese spread (2 T)	3,0 g
Ricotta	3,63 g
Lichten Blanc, low-fat	3,96 g
Lower-fat feta	5,1 g
Medium-fat cheese	
Low-fat cream cheese	6,8 g

In Shape medium-fat cheese	6,9 g
Halloumi	7,26 g
Mozzarella	7,75 g
Lichten Blanc, medium-fat	8,25 g
Edam	8,25 g
Parmesan	8,58 g
Pecorino	9,4 g
Feta	9,4 g
Emmenthaler	9,57 g
Full-cream cheese	
Cream cheese	10 g
Tussers	10,1 g
Gouda	10,2 g
Cheddar	10,5 g
Blue cheese	10,7 g
Mascarpone	17,5 g (very high fat!)

Some surprises again?

Reading and interpreting nutritional labels on products are your only guarantee that you'll be eating lower-fat foods, so make sure you acquaint yourself with this skill (see page 141) and get your dietician to help you with the labels of the foods you love to eat.

Chapter 6

Putting it all together

Now that you know why it's so important to choose wisely when you put food on your plate, let us help you make it simple and practical to eat the low-GI, lower-fat way, every day.

Portion control made easy

Although you probably don't want to hear this, you will have to control food portions to some degree if you want to get slim, and stay slim. That's part of eating smart: eating more than your body needs, even if it's low fat, may help you to maintain your body weight, but it won't necessarily result in weight loss. We do, however, have an easy way for you to learn simple portion control:

No weighing.
No measuring.
No need for specialised scales.
No need for specialised foods.

No eating differently from the rest of your family.

Just simple quantities, using your hands as a guide.

Every meal should consist of mainly low-GI carbohydrates that include a generous quantity of vegetables and/or fruit, a small portion of lean protein and a little "good" fat.

To put this into practice for your *main meal*, follow these six simple steps:

1 Choose a lean protein (e.g. skinned chicken breast, trimmed pork, fish, etc.). Make sure your lean protein portion size is no bigger than the palm of your hand and no more than the thickness of your little finger, and that it doesn't fill more than one quarter of your plate. You can be a bit more generous with fish and chicken.

2 Add a low-GI starch (durum wheat pasta, boiled barley, pearled whole wheat/wheat rice, basmati rice, Tastic rice, sweet potato, etc.) – one portion for women and a double portion for men. Your starch portion should also not fill more than one quarter of your plate.

3 Fill the rest of your plate with low-GI vegetables cooked, or as a salad.

4 Add *one* fat to the meal (olive oil salad dressing, *or* nuts, *or* avocado, *or* olives, *or* peanut butter, *or* a lightly fried protein portion, *or* lite margarine on bread or a roll, *or* cheese sauce, *or* ice cream, etc.).

5 End the meal with a piece of fresh fruit, or add the fruit to the meal (for example, apple sauce with pork roast). Alternatively you can reserve the fruit to take as a snack.

6 Lastly, make sure you drink at least one glass of water every time you eat, i.e. with every meal and every snack. If you never eat between meals, drink one glass of water with each meal and at least one glass of water between meals.

See the section on meal suggestions for breakfast, lunch and supper to see how easy and delicious this can be (page 157).

Portion sizes made easy

Starches

A portion is the amount of cooked starch you can hold in one hand, while running, without the food falling out of your hand. Starches include cooked barley, wheat rice, whole corn, sweet potatoes, baby potatoes with skins, cooked dried beans, lentils, baked beans, soya products, etc.

Raw pasta: One woman's handful of raw pasta is roughly one starch portion when cooked. So, for a family of mom, dad and two children, you would use five handfuls of raw pasta (two for dad).

Cereals: A portion is considered to be 125 ml ($\frac{1}{2}$ C). Give preference to low-GI cereals such as High Fibre Bran, wholewheat Pronutro, Bokomo Maximize, Fine Form Muesli, Nature's Source Low GI Muesli, oat bran, etc.

Bread: One machine-cut slice of bread or three low-GI crackers are usually regarded as a portion.

Fruit

One portion of *fresh fruit* is one piece of fruit, or as much as you can hold in one hand, while running, without the fruit falling out of your hand (such as grapes without the stalk).

Deciduous fruits (e.g. apples, pears, peaches, grapes, nectarines, fresh cherries, plums, apricots, kiwifruit and berries) and citrus fruits (e.g. oranges, naartjies, lemons, grapefruit, etc.) are all low-GI fruits.

Fruit juices have slightly higher GI values than the corresponding fresh fruit, because grape juice is usually added. They're also concentrated sources of carbohydrate, since it takes an average of three fruits to make one glass of fruit juice. It's therefore important to:

◆ Drink small quantities of fruit juices (half a glass, *or* 125ml [$\frac{1}{2}$ C], *or* one wineglass equals one fruit juice portion) and give preference to the lower-GI fruit juices (usually deciduous or citrus fruits, but see GI lists in Section 5 [pages 219 and 229] to be sure).

◆ Higher-GI fruit juices (usually made from tropical fruits) can be taken after sport to prevent the common post-exercise "hypo". Mango or litchi juice would, for instance, be absorbed relatively quickly and thus prevent blood sugar levels from dropping too fast after exercise.

◆ Liqui-Fruit and Ceres now state the GI on the nutritional label, but remember to drink these juices diluted (with rooibos tea, sparkling mineral water or plain water) and in small quantities, even if it is a low GI fruit juice. You shouldn't drink more than half a glass, or 125 ml ($\frac{1}{2}$ C) at a time.

Dried fruits should be taken in small portions only, as they are very concentrated sources of carbohydrate. Always imagine the fruit in its fresh form and eat only as much as you would eat of the fresh fruit. Four dried apricot halves are equivalent to two fresh apricots and will therefore make up one fruit portion.

Vegetables

A portion is the quantity of cooked vegetable that you can hold in one hand, while running, without it falling from your hand. Vegetables include cabbage, cauliflower, broccoli, Brussels sprouts, green beans, etc.

The higher-GI vegetables, i.e. yellow pumpkin, carrots, turnips, parsnips, spinach, marog and beetroot, are best eaten only in combination with other low-GI foods, such as legumes or peas.

Protein

For your *main meal*, the protein portion size should be no larger than the palm of your hand, and the thickness of your little finger. You can be a little more generous with fish and chicken.

The protein portion size for *breakfast* and your *light meal* should be half the size of your main meal portion, i.e. half the size of the palm of your hand and the thickness of your little finger.

Remember to choose only *one* protein food per meal, i.e. either a portion of meat, *or* fish, *or* chicken, *or* egg, *or* cheese, *or* milk, *or* yoghurt, *or* legumes. (Dairy also contains protein, but because it contains calcium as well, it falls in a separate group). Should you choose to eat two types of protein for your main meal – for example, a small chop and feta cheese in your salad – then both the cheese and chop must fit into the palm of your hand. Should you choose to eat two types of protein for your breakfast or light meal – for example, one "matchbox" (30 g) cheese and 125 ml ($^1/_2$ C) cooked dried beans, peas or lentils – both should fit into half the size of the palm of your hand.

Dairy

One small tub (100 ml) low-fat or fat-free yoghurt (sweetened), *or* one tub (175 ml) plain or sugar-free low-fat/fat-free yoghurt, *or* 250 ml (1 C) low-fat or fat-free milk, *or* a "matchbox" piece (30 g) of any lower-fat cheese.

Fats

A portion is generally 5 ml (1 t). The aim is to add only *one* fat to any given meal. This means the salad dressing, *or* the margarine on the roll, *or* the avocado in the salad, *or* the nuts, *or* food fried lightly in 5 ml (1 t) oil or "fake-fried" in 2 ml oil, *or* the low-fat mayonnaise, *or* the low-oil salad cream, *or* the single rasher of streaky bacon (trimmed back bacon is regarded as a protein), *or* a small portion of dessert. (Do remember that most desserts also contain carbohydrates, which means that you'll have to compensate by having less or no starch with your food. See page 45 to learn more about compensating.)

Note: When using commercially bought, ready-to-eat foods such as fish fingers, burger patties, etc., check the nutritional content on the label. The fat content per portion that you're going to eat should be no more than 5 g of fat.

Other tips for low-GI, lower-fat eating

Timesavers

If you're one of those people who never seem to have time to cook a meal from scratch, don't despair. Every supermarket has speciality shelves laden with all sorts of pastes and minced spice and herb mixes that can add instant gourmet flavour to many meals – pastes such as chilli, garlic, ginger, curry, Thai curries, etc. There are also many readymade sauces in pouches, cans, jars and packets. The secret is to use only those that are low in fat. By learning to interpret the nutritional information on food packages, you will be able to shop intelligently and put together low-GI, lower-fat meals in a jiffy.

Using frozen vegetables saves on preparation time and ensures that you'll still have sufficient vegetables with all meals.

In addition, the Glycemic Index Foundation of South Africa (GIFSA) has put together an endorsement logo which guarantees that the products bearing this logo are GI and fat rated. (See Label-reading skills on page 140 for the logos and explanations.)

Suitable drinks

Cooldrinks

Cordials: All artificially sweetened cordials are acceptable, but try not to consume more than *two* glasses of cordial a day, unless you drink no carbonated cold drinks, in which case you can drink a maximum of *four* glasses. It's preferable, however, to drink water, as it aids weight loss.

◆ Brookes Low Cal (all flavours)
◆ Lecol Diet (all flavours)
◆ Sweet-O

Carbonated cooldrinks: All artificially sweetened drinks are acceptable, but try not to consume more than *two* tins (340 ml each) a day, unless you drink no cordials, in which case you can consume a maximum of *four* tins. As before, it's better to drink water, as it aids weight loss.

◆ Tab and other caffeine-free cola drinks. (Note that it's preferable to drink caffeine-free drinks as caffeine may raise blood glucose and blood cholesterol levels, as well as blood pressure.)
◆ Diet Sprite
◆ Sparkling Lemon Lite
◆ Appletizer: The 200 ml size diluted with 200 ml soda water or mineral water and sipped *slowly*. Important: Don't drink more than this, as fruit juice is very concentrated and this quantity is equal to two portions of fruit.
◆ Iced tea (sugar-free)

Water:
◆ Mineral water, still or sparkling
◆ Flavoured mineral waters containing fructose, sorbitol, or lactitol (check labels). Remember that more than 20 g a day of these sweeteners may cause diarrhoea and retinal damage and also adds kilojoules.
◆ Soda water
◆ Filtered water

Dairy drinks are especially good at lunchtime for children who take part in sports during the afternoon. It's important to check that the drink you choose is lower in fat. Check the nutrition table on the label, and make sure that the fat content is 2 g of fat, or less, per 100 ml. Always aim for this fat content in drinks; the international standard for a drink to be truly low fat is 1,5 g per 100 ml, not 3 g per 100 g, as for solids.

- Low-fat drinking yoghurt (all flavours), 200 ml size
- Low-fat flavoured milk (all flavours), 200 ml size
- Low-fat milk, 200 ml – 250 ml ($^4/_5$ – 1 C)
- Low-fat milk, 200 ml ($^4/_5$ C), with Nesquick (10 ml [1 heaped t]).

Note: Do not drink more than one of the above a day.

Hot drinks

Artificial sweeteners may be used if desired, but don't use more than 10 tablets (or 5 sachets) a day.

- Decaffeinated coffee with low-fat or fat-free milk (no sugar)
- "Skinny" cappuccino, decaffeinated (no sugar). This means it's made with low-fat or fat-free milk froth, not whipped cream!
- Low-caffeine tea with low-fat or fat-free milk (no sugar)
- Rooibos tea with low-fat or fat-free milk (no sugar)
- Milo made with low-fat or fat-free milk (10 ml [1 heaped t] Milo in 250 ml [1 C] low-fat milk, no sugar added)
- Horlicks made with low-fat or fat-free milk (10 ml [1 heaped t] Horlicks in 250 ml [1 C] low-fat milk, no sugar added)
- Hot chocolate made with low-fat or fat-free milk (10 ml [1 heaped t] in 250 ml [1 C] milk.) The hot chocolate powder doesn't have to be sugar-free if you're not overweight; blood glucose control will be just as effective if the powder contains sugar, because milk slows down the absorption of sugar. Don't add sugar, however.

Note: It's preferable to use caffeine-free drinks as caffeine may raise blood glucose and blood cholesterol levels, as well as blood pressure.

Alcoholic drinks

Don't consume more than one (for women) or two (for men) alcohol units per day. Alcohol adds extra kilojoules to your daily intake and can therefore jeopardise your weight loss programme. In addition, the human body always prefers to use alcohol as an energy source, rather than fat, so drinking too much alcohol will also diminish fat loss. It's preferable to have your alcoholic drink *with* your meal, as alcohol is absorbed directly from the stomach and may cause hypoglycaemia if taken on an empty stomach.

◆ Dry or "lite" white wine
◆ Dry red wine
◆ Wine "spritzer" (wine mixed with soda water)
◆ Brut (dry) champagne
◆ Dry sherry
◆ "Lite" beer
◆ Rock shandy made with bitters and Diet Sprite
◆ Spirits such as whisky, brandy, vodka, etc. Have a single tot, topped up again and again with soda water, caffeine-free diet cola or Diet Sprite.

Note: One alcohol unit is equal to:
◆ 125ml ($^1/_2$ C) dry wine
◆ 60 ml (1 sherry glass) sherry
◆ 340 ml can "lite" beer
◆ 170 ml ($^1/_2$ can) standard beer
◆ 25 ml (1 tot) spirits
◆ 250 ml (1 C) "spritzer" (at least half should be soda water or ice)
◆ 170 ml ($^1/_2$ can or bottle) apple cider
◆ 113 ml ($^1/_3$ bottle) spirit cooler such as Smirnoff Spin, as they contain both alcohol and sugar.

Reducing the Glycemic Index of your meals

Our modern, eat-on-the-run lifestyle means it's a real challenge to change your mindset and make a determined effort not to eat those high-GI, high-fat foods that beckon to be eaten at every turn. Once you've made up your mind to put into practice the practical tips listed in this chapter, however, you'll be well rewarded with steady weight loss, sustained energy throughout the day and a great sense of achievement.

Sandwiches and rolls: the quickest lunch of all

With almost all bread and rolls being high GI, it becomes very difficult to stick to buying wheat-free rye breads or seed loaves, which generally have a lower GI. What are you going to do when you can only get the high-GI breads and rolls, and there's no time to buy the lower-GI breads?

Simply use the high-GI bread or roll and combine it with low-GI fillings.

Legumes, dried beans, peas and lentils are very effective at lowering the GI of any meal. Using this information to your advantage is the secret of low-GI eating.

As a bonus, legumes contain sterols and sterolins, which actively reduce cholesterol levels. They're also high in fibre and therefore combat constipation, are very filling and even protect against cancer. Legumes are truly a wonder food!

Here are four delicious ways you can add legumes to your meals made with high-GI breads and rolls, thereby lowering the GI of these meals:

◆ Use *hummus* (recipe on page 207) as a thick spread on each slice of bread used in the sandwich, or on each side of your bread roll. (Obviously you would then omit the margarine or butter.) Add lots of salad vegetables and a little lean ham, cheese, tuna or chicken for a delicious, lower-fat and low-GI sandwich or roll.

◆ Mashed baked beans in tomato sauce, used as a thick "relish" on each slice of bread in the sandwich, adds moisture and lots of taste to the filling.

◆ Mashed cooked small white beans, mixed with a little low-fat or lite mayonnaise, makes a perfect margarine substitute for all savoury sandwiches. Mash a whole tin of small white beans or butter beans with equal parts of low-fat mayonnaise, store in an airtight container in the fridge and use on all your sandwiches. It keeps well in the fridge for one week.

◆ One of our favourites is to put three-bean salad (recipe on page 211) on a dry roll, add a small grilled chicken breast, lettuce and lots of other salad vegetables and then really tuck into this rather large "chicken burger". If you don't have chicken, ham or tuna (canned in brine), or any other lean meat can be used instead.

If you don't fancy any one of these suggestions, you can also lower the GI of bread or rolls by drinking a glass of low-fat or fat-free milk, or eating one portion of yoghurt (see portion sizes on page 119) with your meal.

Alternatively, you can add a fruit to your lunch for a good source of antioxidants and to help lower the GI of the meal, unless you want to keep it for an in-between snack.

> ◆ **By using low-GI foods as the main source of carbohydrate in every meal, the GI of the whole meal is effectively reduced.** ◆

Using Legumes
We all have to relearn how to use legumes on a daily basis. The secret is not to make a meal of beans and lentils, but to "hide" the legume within the meal. Buy every kind there is and experiment, adding one kind to every meal, to find out which legumes you like best, and to ensure they're included in every meal. Our low-GI, lower-fat recipe book, *Eating for Sustained Energy* (Tafelberg, 2000) will give you lots of ideas.

Here are some of the ways cooked dried beans and lentils can be added to meals:

Baked beans are the most versatile and tasty of all the ready-to-eat legumes available on supermarket shelves. Although baked beans contain sugar, they're still low GI. Our grocery cupboards are always well stocked with baked beans in tomato sauce, as they are such a wonderful, quick and easy standby.

Here are some of the many uses we've found for baked beans:

◆ On toast, as a light meal or for breakfast.
◆ As a side dish (salad) with any meal. Baked beans would, for example, go very well with a mixed salad, a little lean cold meat, fish or chicken and a fresh rye roll for lunch on a hot summer's day.
◆ Hot baked beans with a traditional English bacon and egg breakfast (lean grilled bacon and one egg, either poached or fried in a pan sprayed with nonstick cooking spray). Add a grilled tomato and mushrooms.
◆ Added to minestrone soup, baked beans in tomato sauce automatically add the tomato flavour and the haricot beans traditionally

125

found in minestrone. Pasta can also be added 15 minutes before serving, unless you prefer to eat bread with your soup.

◆ Add to any stew, casserole or potjiekos.

◆ Add to mince dishes such as lasagne, bobotie, savoury mince or chilli con carne.

◆ As part of three-bean salad (recipe on page 211), mixed with butter beans, green beans and low-oil French dressing.

◆ As a traditional salad to accompany a braai (barbecue). Mix baked beans with green bananas and a little low-fat mayonnaise. This salad is delicious with any meal.

Note: If you suffer from a spastic colon, make sure you mash the beans or chew them very well, as the skins can irritate a sensitive colon.

Butter beans are available dried in packets or ready-to-eat in tins.

◆ Cooked or tinned butter beans are delicious added to salads and stir-fries.

◆ Butter beans can be part of three-bean salad (recipe on page 211) together with green beans and baked beans and a low-oil salad dressing.

◆ Traditionally, they form part of many meat stews such as oxtail or osso bucco. (Just remember to remove the fat from the meat before cooking!)

◆ Mashed, they're easily incorporated into cakes to replace some of the high-GI flour.

Lentils are available ready to eat in tins or dried in packets. There are two types of lentils: *split lentils*, which are orange in colour, and *whole lentils*, which can be green or brown. Whole dried lentils have to be soaked overnight and then boiled for two hours before use; split lentils don't have to be soaked. If you suffer from a spastic colon, use split lentils rather than whole ones.

◆ Split lentils can be added to any meat dish that's simmered in a gravy, such as stews, casseroles and potjiekos. Add 20 ml (1 heaped T) dried split lentils to the meat dish as you add the cooking liquid and simmer for 20 minutes. The lentils soften and disintegrate to thicken the gravy. They lose their orange colour and become creamy white, and don't influence the colour or taste of the sauce or gravy. It is much better to use this as a thickener than to use higher-GI flour, cornflour, soup powder or gravy powder, as lentils help to lower the GI of the meal, increase the fibre content and are more filling. If you often cook in a hurry, or have a fussy family, try always to have some split lentils in water in the fridge. Add some to the meat dish close to the beginning of the cooking process to ensure that nobody notices the lentils – they won't once the dish is cooked as the lentils will disintegrate completely. Add split lentils to all soups, together with barley or pasta.

◆ Whole lentils add a nutty nuance to mince dishes such as bobotie, lasagne, bolognaise, cottage pie, stews, curries, etc.

◆ Whole lentils mixed in equal parts with rice effectively reduce the GI of any rice.

◆ Whole lentils are delicious sprinkled into salads and stir-fries.

◆ Whole lentils can also be sprinkled on sandwich fillings to give an interesting crunch and nutty taste.

◆ Whole lentils can also be sprouted and added to salads or sandwiches.

Split pea dhal is made from yellow split peas that have been soaked overnight and then cooked to form a soft purée, much like sloppy mashed potatoes. Fortunately it's also available ready to eat, in tins.

◆ Add dhal to soups and stews to thicken them.

◆ Pea or lentil dhal can be added to mashed potato, together with a little nutmeg, for an interesting flavour. It will also lower the GI of the mashed potato, which has a high GI value.

Low Glycemic Index starches for main meals

If you're still hesitant about trying to add small quantities of legumes to every meal, you can opt for using the alternative low-GI starches with your meals. Of course, it would be best to use the low-GI starches and also add some beans or lentils to your meal!

Since potatoes and most types of rice (especially "sticky" rice, due to its lower amylose content) have high GI values, you should try to use the low-GI starches listed below instead.

Pearled barley: It's interesting to note that barley is also very effective in lowering cholesterol levels, because it has a high soluble fibre content.

Since barley takes longer to cook than rice, it's best to cook the whole packet (as you would cook rice, only longer), then freeze it in portions and reheat as required.

◆ Serve barley, instead of rice, with meals.

◆ Barley can also be mixed in equal quantities with white or brown rice to effectively lower the GI of the higher-GI rice.

◆ Pearled barley makes a tasty salad mixed with tuna, ham or chicken. Add some chopped vegetables and a low-oil dressing and you'll have a delicious summer lunch. See page 201 for a tasty salad dressing.

Pearled wholewheat, wheat rice or stampkoring: Wheat rice is cooked in exactly the same way as rice, but for a little longer. Like barley, it's more practical to cook the whole packet at once and then freeze it in portions.

◆ Use instead of rice with roasts, curries, chicken and stews.

◆ Mix with barley and/or lentils and use instead of rice.

◆ Use in salads.

Basmati rice: This aromatic rice has a lower GI than ordinary white or brown rice, because it has a higher amylose content. It's available in supermarkets under the label Tasmati Rice (from Tastic). Basmati rice takes slightly longer to cook than ordinary rice.

◆ To date, only the GI of Tastic rice has been tested in South Africa, so it's best to mix other white and brown rice with lentils in a one to one ratio, should you not be able to get basmati or Tastic rice.

◆ Alternatively, pearled barley or pearled wheat can be mixed in equal quantities with white or brown rice to effectively lower the GI of the higher-GI rice, as suggested above.

Sweet potatoes: Because sweet potatoes have a very high soluble fibre content they have a low GI value, which also helps to bind and reduce cholesterol levels.

◆ Baked or microwaved in their skins (prick before baking or microwaving), boiled or even lightly fried in a little olive oil, they make a delicious substitute for potatoes at any meal. (See recipe for roast sweet potato and butternut [page 210]).

◆ Sweet potatoes make a good soup base and can also be roasted.

Pasta: Pasta has to be made from the hard winter wheat called durum wheat. It's so hard that it cannot be ground to flour, and only makes "gritty bits" called semolina. Because of this hardness, pasta made from durum wheat or durum wheat semolina has a low GI value. Pasta bearing the GIFSA Green logo is also low GI.

◆ Always check on the ingredients list that the noodles, macaroni or spaghetti you are about to buy was made from durum wheat or durum wheat semolina.

◆ Homemade pasta is usually made from ordinary flour and will therefore have a high GI value.

Salads and vegetables

Another easy way of reducing the GI of any meal is to add large portions of low-GI vegetables or a large salad with a low-oil dressing, so that the vegetables make up at least half the volume on your plate. Remember that higher-GI vegetables such as carrots, pumpkin, turnips, parsnips, spinach, marog and beetroot must be combined with at least one low-GI food, such as dried beans. Contrary to popular belief, vegetables and salads are the most filling foods you can eat. They also help you slim, because they don't contain many kilojoules and your body has to work to digest them.

Baking

Baked goods offer their own special challenges as the main ingredient in any cake, biscuit, muffin, scone, bread, rusk, tart, etc. is high-GI cake flour. The secret to lowering the GI of baked products is to substitute as much of the flour as is practical with another low-GI starch source: Unfortunately, you can't replace all the flour, because you'd end up with muesli!

◆ Mashing a whole tin of drained beans and adding it to a batter allows you to leave out one third to half the flour called for in the original recipe. You will also have to adjust the quantity of liquid called for in the recipe (it's usually less). For recipes adjusted this way, see *Eating for Sustained Energy*.

◆ Using low-fat or skimmed milk, or low-fat or fat-free yoghurt, as the liquid in a batter also helps to lower the GI of the cake or other batter.

◆ Adding one or two freshly grated apples to batter not only allows you to leave out some of the flour, but also to omit at least half the fat (oil, margarine or butter) and some of the sugar called for in the recipe. For recipes adjusted this way, see the recipe section of this book.

◆ One of the easiest ways of lowering the GI of a baked product is to use oat bran or lower-GI oats in place of some of the flour called for in the recipe. Oat bran is the fibre of oats in its pure form. Not only are oats and oat bran lower GI, they're also very effective at reducing cholesterol levels. When baking, you can very successfully substitute oat bran for *one third to half* the flour called for. Bake as usual. Oat bran is very good in muffins, banana bread, Christmas cake, rusks, crumpets, pancakes and scones. To get your family used to oat bran, start by substituting oat bran for one quarter of the flour and gradually work your way up to substituting oat bran for a third (but not more than half) the quantity of flour called for in the recipe.

Remember to add a little more of the raising agent (baking powder, bicarbonate of soda or yeast), when substituting lower-GI ingredients for the flour.

Here are some ways to add oat bran to meals:
◆ Oat bran is delicious added to fruit yoghurt.
◆ Add oat bran to muesli.
◆ Add raw oat bran (15 ml – 45 ml [1 – 3 T] per serving) to cooked mealiemeal, Maltabella, oats and Taystee Wheat porridge, after cooking – simply stir into the porridge.
◆ Oat bran makes a delicious porridge on its own or mixed with oats, but it's best eaten raw or added to cooked oats.

Fruit (fresh)

As a general rule, fruits are suitable for stabilising blood sugar levels, but there is one exception: *All melons* (including watermelon, sweet melon and "spanspek") have high GI values, and should never be eaten on their own. Always combine them in meals containing low-GI foods:
◆ Baked beans on toast and sweet melon for dessert.
◆ Spanspek followed by High Fibre Bran with low-fat milk (and a little sugar, if desired).

Tropical fruits such as mango, banana, pineapple, litchis and pawpaw all have intermediate GI values, which means that they're absorbed within the space of about two hours. Always combine them with other low-GI foods.

◆ Banana, cut into All-bran Flakes with low-fat milk (and an optional sprinkling of sugar).

◆ Vegetable soup containing lots of legumes, together with seed loaf and a fruit salad made from pawpaw, banana, oranges and apples.

Citrus and deciduous fruits all have low-GI values.

◆ The more tart (sour) a fruit, the lower its GI value.

◆ Citrus fruits include: Oranges, naartjies, grapefruit, lemons and minneolas.

◆ Deciduous fruits include: Apricots, plums, fresh cherries, apples, pears, peaches, nectarines, grapes (watch portions), kiwifruit, granadillas, strawberries and other berries.

◆ Apples and pears, freshly grated and added to cake and other batters, not only lower the GI of the baked product, but also help to retain moisture in the mixture and so enable you to use less fat in the recipe.

See pages 118 and 119 for a discussion of fruit juices and dried fruit.

Jams and marmalade
Homemade plum, apricot or berry jam and marmalade have lower GI values because of the higher fruit concentration and acidity, and are quite safe to use in small quantities (not more than 10 g [2 level t] per meal). All Fine Form jams and sugar-free jams have low GI values.

Low-GI tips for emergencies

You're at a dinner party, out shopping, or at a friend's house, and the food on your plate isn't within your control. What do you do?

Here are some easy ways to reduce the GI (and fat content) of everyday meals:

◆ Add a low-GI fruit to your meal as a starter or pudding.

◆ Add low-fat or fat-free yoghurt (fruit or plain) to the meal as your dessert or as a protein.

◆ Add a glass of low-fat or skimmed milk to the meal.

◆ Add three-bean salad (recipe on page 211) or baked beans to your plate of food.

◆ Add raw salad vegetables to your meal, even if it's a sandwich.

◆ Add a small glass of low-GI fruit juice, such as orange or apple juice, to your meal. It definitely helps to prevent that sleepy feeling after a high-GI meal.

See page 151 for tips on lowering the GI and fat content of a restaurant or hotel meal, or cocktail party snacks.

Fat-proofing your meals

There are many quick and easy ways to ensure that your everyday meals are lower in fat. It's quite amazing how much difference even a small change can make. Read through the following information and tips and try to implement at least one every day, until it becomes second nature for you to do so.

Fake-frying

Some foods have to be fried to make the most of their flavour. If you have to fry a food, learn to fake-fry it! Pour a little good-quality oil into a frying pan. Heat until the oil is hot and very liquid, but not smoking. Pick up the pan and swirl the oil around to cover the base. *Pour all the oil out of the pan.* You don't have to throw it away, but don't use it over and over. Now *fake-fry* the food in the oil remaining in the pan.

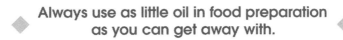

◆ **Always use as little oil in food preparation**
as you can get away with. ◆

Use *top-quality* oils that have maximum nutritional value. These include:

- Cold-pressed olive oil (preferably extra-virgin)
- Canola oil
- Palm oil (Carotino oil), which is bright orange in colour.

Both coconut and palm kernel oil are high in saturated fats and should be avoided. Rather use *palm oil* – which is bright orange and not the same thing as palm kernel oil – as it has a good mono-unsaturated fat content and is full of beneficial antioxidants. It's sold as Carotino oil in South Africa. *Olive oil* and *canola oil* are also good-quality oils (mainly mono-unsaturated) to use in small quantities for cooking.

Watch for hidden fats in:

Muffins
Cakes
Croissants
Scones
Rusks
Savoury crackers
Biscuits
Pâté and spreads
Instant sauces
Popcorn
Crisps
Chips
Chocolates
Health bars

Instant soups
Creamed soups
Tinned soups
Salad dressings
Mayonnaise
Cream dressings
Pies
PastriesSnack bars
Slimming bars
Toasted muesli
Coffee creamers
Milkshakes
Cappuccino with cream

The fat content of some nutritious plant foods needs to be taken into consideration. Look at the table on the next page and you'll see what we mean.

Food	Fat per 100 g	Fat per usual serving
Avocado	15 g	1/2 avocado contains 15g fat
Olives	10,7 g	5 olives contain about 2,5 to 5 g fat (22 small olives = 100 g)
Nuts	50 g+	one handful contains 25 g fat, so beware!
Seeds	30 g+	one handful contains 15 g fat

The following portion sizes are therefore recommended to keep fat within the recommended fat *per meal* (see page 111).

Use only *one* of these per meal:

Food	Portion	Fat content
Avocado	30 g (1 slice)	5 g
Nut	10 g – 20 g	5 g – 10 g
Olives	5 large or 10 small	5 g
Seeds	20 g – 30 g	5 g – 10 g

Did you know?
Lite margarine (10 ml [2 t]) contains 5 g fat
Standard margarine (10 ml [2 t]) contains 8,2 g fat
Butter (10 ml [2 t]) contains 8,2 g fat

Low-oil salad cream, e.g. Trim (10 ml [2 t]) contains 1 g fat
Low-fat mayonnaise, e.g. Hellmann's Lite (10 ml [2 t]) contains 2,5 g fat
Standard mayonnaise (10 ml [2 t]) contains 5 g fat
Fat-reduced cream (10 ml [2 t]) contains 2 g fat
Pouring cream (10 ml [2 t]) contains 4 g fat
Whipping cream (10 ml [1 heaped t]) contains 5 g fat

Did you know?
One pat of foil-covered butter or margarine served in a restaurant contains 10 ml (2 t) butter or margarine. This contains 8 g of fat, which makes it really unnecessary to butter the high-GI roll, considering the higher fat meal you're about to eat. It would be even better

if you didn't eat the roll and butter. Remember, in particular, not to spread butter or margarine on muffins, scones and croissants, which already contain butter, margarine or oil (unlike bread rolls, which contain a minimum of fat).

When making *sandwiches* or eating toast, don't butter the bread or toast automatically. Most of the time there's no need to use butter or margarine; many toppings taste just as good without the added fat. This is especially true if you have a high-fat spread such as peanut butter, avocado, liver pâté, cream cheese spreads, cheese spreads, etc., on your bread. Use only the topping and lose the margarine or butter. If you're using fat-free cottage cheese, you may have a little lite tub margarine.

Do you know how much fat there is in some *common snacks*? Take a closer look at this table and you may be surprised.

Fat content of some common snack foods		
High fat products are marked with an asterisk (*) and very high fat products with two asterisks (**)		
Snack foods	**Portion size**	**Fat per portion**
Chocolate	100 g slab	36 g**
Chocolate bar	one standard bar	10 g –12 g*
Toffees, traditional	one toffee	4 g
Toffees, e.g. Choc éclair	one Choc éclair	0,65 g
Toffees, traditional	200 g packet	40 g**
Fudge	4 cm square (40 g)	5 g
Nougat	15 g piece (1 small)	3 g
Ice cream	100 g (1 C)	16 g**
Ice cream sauce	2 T	20 g**
Soft-serve ice cream	one large	13 g*
Sorbet	100 g (1 C)	8,7 g*
Low-fat ice cream (3% fat)	100 g (1 C)	3 g
Fat-free ice cream (< 0,5% fat, e.g. Dialite)	1 C	0,2 g
Caramel-covered popcorn	45 g packet	1,1 g
Cheese curls	16 g packet	5 g
Crisps, potato	30 g packet	10,8 g*
Crisps, potato (thick cut)	45 g packet	16,12 g**

Crisps, corn	50 g packet (Fritos)	18 g**
Crisps, corn	40 g packet (Nik Naks)	14 g*
Pretzels, plain salted	45 g packet	3 g
Pretzels, thin and lite	45 g packet	2 g
Pretzels, flavoured	45 g packet	7 g – 10 g, depending on flavour*
Chips, hot	200 g (one small serving)	32 g**
Peanuts	55 g packet	27,5 g**

Use the *paper test* to check the fat content of foods you're not sure of (especially in restaurants). Imagine the food on a piece of paper. If it leaves a fat mark on the paper, it's too fatty and shouldn't be eaten.

Choosing the right meat cut

Always use the *leanest cuts of red meat* and stick to small portions (maximum 120 g a person), unless eating out in a restaurant, when ladies' portions should be chosen (150 g cooked weight). Try not to eat red meat more than three times a week.

Leaner beef cuts
    Topside
    Minced topside
    Silverside
    Rump (fat trimmed)
    Veal
Leaner venison
    Ostrich
    Venison
Leaner lamb cuts
    Leg of lamb (fat trimmed)
    Shoulder of lamb (fat trimmed)
Leaner pork cuts
    Ham
    Kassler rib, trimmed of all fat

To keep saturated fats within healthy limits, favour fish and chicken, each of which you should preferably eat twice a week. Red meat should be eaten three times a week – maximum! Alternatively, you can substitute one of your fish or chicken meals with legumes, which contain no fat. Be careful not to add a lot of high-fat ingredients such as cheese, oil, cream and eggs.

To reduce the fat content of *sausages*, either place in hot water to heat, grill under a hot grill or braai over the fire, pricking the skin to release the fat as much as possible. Alternatively, you can opt for lower-fat sausages such as chicken sausage (10% fat) or pork bangers (15% fat), but still cook them in water.

Remember:
◆ The drier the meat, the leaner it is, so topside, aitchbone and venison (including ostrich) are very lean.
◆ Chicken: Avoid the skin, wings and parson's nose as they contain the most fat. Skinned turkey is also a tasty, lean option.
◆ Pork: Cut off all visible fat. The actual meat is rather dry and therefore very lean.
◆ Beef: Fillet, rump and roast beef are reasonably lean. Use topside mince or extra trim/lean mince. See the table on page 112.
◆ Lamb and mutton: Eat occasionally. Cut off all visible fat and skim fat off the gravy. Try grilling the meat and place a pan below to catch the fat, instead of grilling the meat in its own fat. Lamb and mutton contain a lot of hidden (marbled) fat!

The *preparation method* of the protein dish greatly influences the fat content of the meal.

All fish, chicken (without skin) and meat (fat trimmed) should be grilled, baked or roasted without adding any extra oil, lard or other fat during cooking. For tasty recipes, see the Recipe Section.

For stews, casseroles and potjiekos, the meat, fish or chicken should be added *with* the other ingredients, not fried and browned beforehand, unless you fake-fry it. Add beans to reduce the GI of the meal. Use baby potatoes, with skin, instead of chopped potatoes; regard this as the starch in your meal, or use half a portion of rice to compensate for the potatoes in the dish.

Stir-fries are tasty, nutritious and low in fat. Use 5 ml (1 t) of oil to gently brown the meat and onions, add the vegetables and legumes and then some liquid (water, wine, etc.) to steam the dish, rather than fry it. Thicken with a little cornflour mixed with an equal quantity of oat bran or split lentils.

Do *not* use extra oil if the vegetables start to burn; add liquid instead. Add butter beans or lentils to reduce the GI of the meal even more.

Fat-proofing convenience foods

Frozen, crumbed or battered fish, meat or chicken is already fried. Bake on paper towels, without adding extra oil or other fat, to try to render as much fat as possible. Only buy those products that have less than 5 g fat per portion. By law, a product needs to contain at least 30% less fat to be called "Lite", but unfortunately some companies get away with a much smaller reduction in fat. The only way to know whether a product is truly low-fat or lower in fat, is to analyse the label (see Label-reading Skills [page 141]).

Alternatively you can grill the fish, meat or chicken, using non-stick cooking spray, or you can fake-fry it.

In restaurants always ask for a sauce, salad dressing, sour cream, etc. to be served separately so that you can add 5 ml – 10 ml (1 – 2 t) sauce to your food and not drown it in a high-fat sauce.

Choose tinned fish such as tuna and salmon in brine, not oil, or in a tomato or chilli sauce. Check the oil content very carefully. It should be 3 g fat or less per 100 g, but no more than 10 g fat or less per 100 g, or a maximum of 5 g fat per portion.

Fat-proofing bacon and egg breakfasts

The recommended intake of eggs is three per week, i.e. one every second day. Traditional egg and bacon breakfasts are therefore quite in order as long as you grill the bacon (trimmed), and fry the egg in a pan sprayed with nonstick cooking spray or fake-fry it; grill the tomato, poach the mushrooms in a little low-fat milk and eat with seed loaf or rye toast. Add hot baked beans to reduce the GI of the breakfast, and fresh fruit for good nutrition, unless you want to reserve the fruit for an in-between snack.

What a feast!

Salads can be fat traps!

Croutons, avocado, nuts, seeds, olives, mayonnaise and salad dressings are all loaded with fat. Drizzle about 5 ml (1 t) of the salad dressing over the salad – don't drown it – and add only *one* of the fats listed per meal. (See page 117 for portion sizes.)

Baking

When baking, always use at least 50 g ($^{1}/_{4}$ C) less margarine, butter or oil than is called for in the recipe. If you add a grated apple to the batter, you will not only be able to reduce the fat even more, but you'll also be reducing the GI of the batter, not to mention adding fibre, vitamins and minerals. You can even decrease the quantity of sugar in the batter, as apples add quite a bit of sweetness to baking.

Saving fat in milks

Use low-fat milk (2%) for everyday use or a half-and-half mixture of low-fat and skimmed (fat-free) milk, which brings you to milk containing 1% fat. The low-fat milk masks the taste of the skimmed milk, making it less noticeable and more acceptable. Use UHT skimmed milk (in cartons) to make custard, milktart, and white and cheese sauces. Even powdered skimmed milk tastes fine in cooking and baking, especially if you add a little vanilla essence.

Fat-proofing pizzas

Pizzas are a safer choice, as long as they're not drowned in garlic oil (as opposed to fresh garlic) or other high-fat toppings, such as salami, pepperoni, mince, bacon, olives, avocado, etc. Rather choose pizzas topped with ham, chicken, mozzarella cheese and vegetables (tomatoes, onions, mushrooms, etc.), which are low in fat. Regina pizza is a good example. Don't use too much pineapple, as it has a higher GI value.

Remember that the base (crust) is high-GI – balance this with lots of low-GI vegetables, such as tomato, onion, green peppers, asparagus and/or mushrooms, as the topping. Add three-bean salad or a small apple juice and you will successfully reduce the GI of the whole meal – unless, of course, you're eating it after exercise, in which case you need not add the low-GI foods to your meal.

Fat-proofing hamburgers

To reduce the fat and GI of hamburgers effectively, you should make your own patties, using topside mince, and bind the mince with lower-GI oats or oat bran. Then grill the patties without adding any extra oil or other fat, unless you fake-fry them. Slip the patties on to unbuttered rolls. Spread the rolls with mashed baked beans as the "relish" for the hamburger. Lastly, add a good helping of salad, containing lots of veggies (and a low-GI apple), to further reduce the GI of the rolls.

Fat-proofing a toasted sandwich

Lightly spread one side of a slice of seed loaf or wheat-free rye bread with lite tub margarine. Add a little lower-fat cheese, tuna in brine, or chicken with lite mayonnaise. Remember to leave out the margarine if you're using mayonnaise. Spray a snackwich maker with nonstick cooking spray and "toast" your sandwich as dry as possible. If you'd rather use ordinary brown bread, which is high GI, add mashed baked beans to the filling or serve with a salad containing butter beans or baked beans, or at least have a low-GI fruit with your sandwich, to ensure a lower-GI meal.

Quiches are healthy? Think again!

Most bought quiches are made with lots of cream, full-cream milk, full-fat cheeses, fried onions and other vegetables and there's lots of fat in the pastry. For this reason they're very high in fat, and because of the flour in the pastry, they're usually high GI as well.

An average slice of quiche contains at least 30 g of fat, similar to a rich ice cream on a stick or a meat pie.

Quiches should be made with plain low-fat or fat-free yoghurt and low-fat or fat-free milk, instead of cream. Grill the bacon; poach the mushrooms in a little milk and use mozzarella or any other lower-fat cheese. Add any low-GI vegetables, especially legumes, to the filling. Cooked dry beans (instead of tinned) taste like nuts in a quiche. The base should be made with half flour, half oat bran, and as little margarine as possible, preferably lite margarine. For an adapted recipe see our low-GI, lower-fat recipe book, *Eating for Sustained Energy*.

Label-reading skills

Foods are attractively labelled to catch the attention of potential and sometimes unwary buyers and to create a desire to buy that particular product. Little attention is given to the nutritional benefits (or lack of them) of the food. Nutritional information is printed on labels as a secondary function, and only because it is required by law. For this reason the nutritional information is often difficult to find. It's usually on the side panel or on the back of the packaging, in rather small print.

Words such as *diet, slimmers' choice, low-fat, 99% fat-free, sugar-free, diabetic, lite,* and *low-calorie* or *low-kilojoule* often mislead us into thinking the products bearing these labels are "healthy". Healthy for whom? Maybe not for you! You need to learn to be a little more discerning, because products aren't always what they seem to be.

Lite could mean light in colour, light in salt, lighter in fat, lighter in flavour, lighter in energy, in fact, lighter in anything the manufacturer wishes, although, by law, a product is only allowed to be labelled "lite" if the fat content is at least 30% less than that in its standard counterpart. Unfortunately, some companies get away with this.

A good example is "lite" olive oil. It's light in colour and flavour, which means, in fact, that it's more refined and *not* healthier than the darker, less processed olive oils. There's no such a thing as "lite" or low-fat oil; if it's lower in fat it means that some of the fat has been replaced with something that's fat-free, such as water. And if water is added to oil, it will spatter in the frying pan, resulting in a mess in your kitchen.

Another example is "Lite" crisps, which probably weigh less, but don't contain less fat per 100 g or portion, so *check the labels!* We cannot emphasise this enough.

Something that's claimed to be *80% fat-free* may, in fact, not be low-fat at all. What it really means is that the product contains 20% fat. A lower-fat cheese, for example, is labelled 80% fat-free, but this means it still contains 20 g of fat per 100 g, or 6,9 g of fat per "matchbox" (30 g) portion – not low-fat at all, merely lower in fat than standard hard cheeses. For the fat content of various cheeses, see page 114.

Another sneaky claim is *reduced by [say] 30% fat*. Reduced from what level (in the first place), and, secondly, does the reduction make sense? As an example, take Gouda cheese that's reduced by 30% fat. On average, cheese contains 30% fat, so a 30% reduction would mean that this particular Gouda cheese still contains 20% fat, and in order to be classed as a truly low-fat cheese it should not contain more than 3 g of fat per 100 g (3% fat). This doesn't mean that the fat reduction is insignificant; any reduction is better than no reduction at all, but the implication to the unwary consumer is that it is "healthy" and can therefore be eaten in unlimited quantities, which is simply not true.

Cholesterol-free or *low cholesterol* may well mean that the food in question is low in cholesterol, but it can still be a high-fat food, and even be high in saturated fats, which raise cholesterol levels. Remember that no plant food can contain cholesterol, since plants cannot manufacture it. This means that, while all plant oils are cholesterol-free, they're still 100% fat, and therefore high-fat foods, regardless of the type of oil. In fact, some "cholesterol-free" oils, such as palm kernel oil and coconut oil, are very high in saturated fats and promote the formation of "bad" LDL cholesterol in the body.

The "cholesterol-free" label does *not* imply that an oil can be used liberally. For optimum health, *all* oils should be used in minute quantities. See page 133 for a discussion of the better types of oils and fats to use.

Often the term "cholesterol-free" also appears on the labels of fruit juices. This is clearly nonsense, and misleading, as no fruit juice contains cholesterol.

Sugar-free. This old-time favourite implies that the sugar-free food can be eaten in huge quantities as it is inherently "healthier", merely by virtue of the fact that it is sugar-free. The fact that a product claims to be sugar-free means simply that it doesn't contain any added sucrose (table sugar). It can still, however, contain large quantities of glucose under the guise of dextrose, maltose or maltodextrin. All of these are much more harmful to blood glucose and insulin control than sugar, as they have a GI of 100 or more and will therefore raise the GI of the product much more than sugar does! Other sugars that could be added to the product include fructose, lactose, grape juice concentrate, sorbitol, lactitol, maltitol, etc., all of which add to the energy (kilojoule) content of the food. Grape juice, in fact, has the same GI as sugar (i.e. 65), which means that jams containing "pure grape juice and no added sugar" are no better for blood glucose control than those which contain sugar, unless, of course, less grape juice is used. Many "sugar-free" products have a high GI value and are often high in fat to boot, especially in the case of baked products. This is particularly true of those sweetened with intense sweeteners such as aspartame, cyclamates and saccharine. Sorbitol, lactitol, maltitol and fructose add kilojoules to the product and can cause retinal damage (in the case of fructose) or gastrointestinal upset (in the case of the other three).

◆ **Reading the labels of these products is imperative.
Don't fall into the high-GI, high-fat trap.** ◆

Products that are labeled *diabetic* are based on the old premise that diabetic diets only need to be sugar-free. They're usually only free of sucrose, have no fat restriction at all and, more often than not, have a higher fat content than the standard product. The most disconcerting part, however, is that most of these products are very high GI, and definitely not suitable for slimmers, let alone diabetics, as they often contain high-GI sugars such as glucose, maltose, dextrose and/ or maltodextrins. A good example here is diabetic biscuits, which are higher in fat than standard biscuits and are also high-GI – most unsuitable for slimmers and diabetics. To be absolutely sure that a product is low-GI and low-fat or lower fat, look for the green GIFSA logos of the Glycemic Index Foundation of South Africa. These logos are in the process of being phased in, and will replace the Jack Spratt logos currently seen on tested products. Please see page 217 for the colour logos.

The GIFSA Green Plus logo means that the product or food endorsed with this logo is low in fat (3 g fat or less per 100 g food) and has a low GI value (40 or lower).

The GIFSA Green logo means that the product or food endorsed with this logo is lower in fat (3,1 g to 10 g fat per 100 g food) and has a low GI value (55 or lower).

The GIFSA Orange logo means that the product or food endorsed with this logo is lower in fat than its standard counterpart, and has an intermediate GI (69 or lower). The fat is always controlled to a maximum of 15 g per 100 g food.

The GIFSA Red logo means that the product or food endorsed with this logo is lower in fat than its standard counterpart and has a high GI (70 and above). The fat is always controlled to a maximum of 15 g per 100 g food.

The *Heart Foundation mark* can only be displayed on those products that have applied for endorsement by the South African Heart Foundation. These products will be low, or sometimes lower, in fat, low or lower in saturated fat and low in sodium. This mark, however, does not give any indication of the GI of the product. In addition, there are many products on the market that would fall into this category (low-fat, low saturated fat and low sodium), but haven't applied for endorsement, and therefore do not display the Heart Foundation mark.

The *Weighless mark* indicates that a product is energy (kilojoule or calorie) controlled. By default, most of these products are lower in fat, but not necessarily low in fat, saturated fat or sodium. As with the Heart Mark, this mark does not give any indication of the GI of the product. Unfortunately, many of the foods bearing this mark are, in fact, high GI.

If you check for the green GIFSA logos, you can be sure that the product is indeed lower in fat and has a low GI value.

As many products do not carry any endorsement marks at all, you need to learn how to interpret the nutritional information on products.

Nutritional label interpretation involves three main processes:
1. Determining how much fat is contained in 100 g of the product and in one portion.
2. Determining the type of fat in the product.
3. Determining the Glycemic Index of the product.

The simple, step-by-step method outlined below will enable you to assess the nutritional information you'll find on the packaging of most foods, quickly and accurately.

Know what you're eating

Read the label to determine the fat content and assess the Glycemic Index of the food.

Here's a step-by-step guide to nutritional label reading.
1. Check the total weight of the product.
2. Estimate how much of the product would be a portion for you, using as a guideline the portion sizes given on the pack. Turn to the small print on the side or back panel, where the nutritional information is.
3. The nutritional information is always given per 100 g of product. Look up how many grams of fat are in 100 g of the product.
4. You now have the quantity of fat in 100 g. The next question is: What is your portion size? Is it 100 g, or twice that quantity, i.e. 200 g? Or is it 50 g (half), or 25 g (quarter)? Or anything else? Remember to multiply or divide accordingly. If, for example, a product is 3% fat or 3 g fat per 100 g of food, a 50 g portion will contain 1,5 g fat. If your portion size is 500 g, as would be the case with lasagne, it will contain 15 g fat, which is higher than the maximum quantity of fat one ladies meal should contain. You have now established the amount of fat per portion.
5. Ideally, the fat content per portion should fall between *3 g and 5 g of fat per portion for women and up to 7 g of fat per portion for men.* See How much fat is healthy? (pages 109).
6. The *type* of fat is also important. To check this, look at the ingredients, which are listed in order of quantity used, by mass (weight) from highest to lowest.
7. The ingredients listed below are all sources of saturated fats (bad fats):

milk solids, milk, cheese, butter, cream, lard, marine fat (often used in processed foods such as cheap margarine), hydrogenated vegetable fat, eggs, meat, chicken.

8. Any ingredients high in saturated fats listed as one of the first three ingredients will tell you that the fat in the product is mostly saturated fat. Ideally, this saturated fat should be no more than half, but preferably only one third of the total fat content.

9. Now check the Glycemic Index (GI) of the product. Again, look at the ingredients listed.

10. The ingredients listed below indicate high GI ingredients:

◆ Flour (wheat, cake, bread, potato, rice, Nutty Wheat, cornflour)
◆ Modified starch
◆ Starch
◆ Maltodextrin
◆ Maltose
◆ Dextrose
◆ Glucose
◆ Pasta (unless specified as made from durum wheat or durum wheat semolina)
◆ Potatoes
◆ Pumpkin
◆ Rice
◆ Breadcrumbs

11. Any one of these high-GI carbohydrates, listed as one of the first three ingredients, indicates that the product is probably high GI.

Let's look at an example: You pick up a box of frozen spinach and feta pies. They should be "healthy" you say to yourself, as spinach is a vegetable, which is fat-free and healthy. Fortunately, before you drop them into your trolley, you decide to assess the nutritional merits of the pies.

The box of pies weighs 600 g and contains four individual pies, so one pie weighs 150 g, which should be enough for a portion, especially for women. You decide you'll have one pie, with a salad, for your lunch.

The nutritional information, in small print on one of the sides of the packaging, reads as follows:

Typical nutritional information per 100 g product:
Protein 7,0 g
Fat 16,0 g
Carbohydrates 17,0 g
Energy 973 kJ
Ingredients: Pastry: Wheat flour, vegetable and/or marine fat, water, salt
Filling: Full-cream milk, spinach, Cheddar cheese, water, onion, egg, vegetable fat, modified starch, wheat flour, Feta cheese, garlic, spices, salt

You now check the nutritional information box to find out how much fat there is in 100 g of pie, and find that it's 16 g fat per 100 g, which is more than the recommended quantity. The pie you wish to eat, however, weighs 150 g, so the fat content per portion is 16 x 1,5 = 24 g fat! This is way over the recommendation of less than 5 g fat per portion or 10 g – 13 g per meal for women and 7 g per portion or 13 g – 17 g per meal for men. So you'll have to put down this particular box of pies and find another with a lower fat content.

Looking at the ingredients list, you'll see that *vegetable/marine fat* is the second ingredient in the pastry, and *full-cream milk* and *Cheddar cheese* are among the first three ingredients in the filling. From this you can conclude that the fats in these pies are mostly saturated fat. In terms of your cancer and heart disease risk, these pies are definitely a poor choice – and a disastrous choice for slimmers! (Read "Sorting out beneficial and detrimental fats" [page 108].)

Now you look at the GI of these pies. Check the list of ingredients for high-GI items in the pastry and the filling. Wheat flour is the first ingredient in the pastry, which makes this very high GI. One could always eat half the pastry and all the filling, however, as the filling contains less of the higher-GI ingredients. You could also add a little extra salad which contains low-GI ingredients such as beans, in order to compensate for the high-GI flour. Modified starch and wheat flour are both high-GI ingredients in the filling, but aren't among the first three ingredients, so the filling should have a lower GI value. The very high fat content totally rules out this product for your lunch, however, especially if you want to lose weight and are trying to be health conscious. Alternatively, you could compensate by eating fat-free foods for the rest of the day, as you consumed almost all the fat for an entire day in one meal. Do remember that it would be much healthier to eat "good fats" than all the bad fats in this pie.

Go to your grocery cupboard, fridge or freezer right now and take out any product you like. Follow the step-by-step guide to label interpretation and see how the product fares:

◆ How much fat does it contain per 100 g and per portion?
◆ Does it contain mainly saturated or unsaturated fat?
◆ How does it rate on the Glycemic Index?

Low-GI, lower-fat foods to keep in your fridge or freezer

Note: If you want specific brand names, you can look them up in the GI lists at the back of this book or in the *SA GI Guide*, available from GIFSA (www.gifoundation.com).

◆ Low-fat or fat-free fruit yoghurt (sweetened or unsweetened)
◆ Low-fat or fat-free plain yoghurt to use in salad dressings, in baking, and instead of cream in sauces
◆ Low-fat or fat-free milk, or both
◆ Low-fat or fat-free cottage cheese (5 g fat or less per 100 g)
◆ Creamed or medium-fat cottage cheese, to use instead of cream cheese (10 g fat or less per 100 g)
◆ Low-fat cheese spread and wedges
◆ Lower-fat cheeses, e.g. Lichten Blanc, In Shape, mozzarella, low-fat feta, etc.
◆ Low-fat, fat-free or lite ice cream
◆ Low-oil or oil-free salad dressings
◆ Salad vegetables, e.g. tomatoes, lettuce, cucumber, celery, cabbage, etc.
◆ Fresh and frozen vegetables for steaming or microwaving, or to use in soups, e.g. broccoli, cauliflower, green beans, baby marrows, patty pans, gem squash, brinjals, etc.
◆ Gherkins and other pickles
◆ Peppadews
◆ Deciduous fruits: apples, apricots, pears, peaches, nectarines, plums, kiwifruit, fresh cherries, etc.
◆ Citrus fruits: oranges, lemons, naartjies, grapefruit, limes, etc.

◆ Low-GI fruit juices (see the GI list at the back of this book as well as Portion control [page 118] as fruit juices are very concentrated)
◆ Sweet potatoes
◆ Corn on the cob (mealies)
◆ Low-GI oats (see the GI list at the back of the book for lower-GI options)
◆ Oat bran (keep in the fridge, as insects know which foods are healthy and go for them)
◆ Wheat germ (a rich source of vitamin E, it can be added to cereals and baking. Keep in the fridge for the same reason as in the case of oats and oat bran.)
◆ Digestive bran (very good for the digestive system; add to porridges, muffins, etc.)
◆ Low-GI jams (see the GI list at the back of this book)
◆ Artificially sweetened cooldrinks such as Tab, Lemon Lite, Diet Sprite, etc. instead of Coke, Fanta, etc.
◆ Sliced ham, silverside, pastrami, smoked beef, smoked chicken (all lower-fat cold meats), as well as ground biltong
◆ Lower-fat processed meat such as lower-fat, lower-salt Viennas, Russians, polony and bacon
◆ Lower-fat sausages such as chicken sausage, pork bangers
◆ Skinned chicken, topside mince, ostrich steaks and kebabs
◆ Hake, kingklip and trout fillets
◆ Extra Lite crumbed fish

Low-GI, lower-fat foods to keep in your grocery cupboard or pantry

Note: For specific brand names, check the GI lists at the back of this book or look in the *SA GI Guide*, available from GIFSA (www.gifoundation.com).

- Fat-free milk powder
- Three-bean salad: can, jar or stand-up pouch
- Curried beans (kerrieboontjies)
- Canned green beans
- Canned mushrooms
- Canned asparagus
- Tomato purée, paste and chopped tomato (canned)
- Baked beans
- Lentils, canned or dried
- Small white beans, canned or dried
- Butter beans, canned or dried
- Split lentils, dried
- Dried low-GI fruits e.g. pears, apples, apricots, peaches, prunes and sultanas
- Canned fruit in fruit juice, e.g. apples, apricots, pears and fruit salad
- Lower-GI oats
- Whole-wheat Pronutro, Original or Apple Bake
- High Fibre Bran or Pick 'n Pay Shredded Bran
- Maximize cereal
- Oat bran
- Fine Form muesli
- Nature's Source low-GI muesli
- Provita, Original and Multigrain
- Bran crispbread
- Pearled barley
- Wheat rice, stampkoring, pearled wholewheat
- Basmati rice and Tastic rice
- Pasta made from durum wheat/durum wheat semolina or those marked with the GIFSA logo
- Low-GI jams
- Sugar-free cordials
- Sustagen
- Soya flour

- Low-GI bread, e.g. seed loaf and wheat-free rye bread
- Cape Seed Loaf bread mix. Add yoghurt or *low-fat* buttermilk, a few spoonfuls of oat bran, as well as an apple to this bread mix for a delicious low-GI bread.

Eating out: finding your way around the menu

The beauty of the low-GI, lower-fat nutrition plan is that you can, with a little forethought, eat out in restaurants or elsewhere without worrying about not being able to find low-GI, low-fat menu items that are both tasty and exciting. Read through the tips that follow and make a note of those you wish to use next time you eat out. You'll be amazed at the sense of achievement you'll feel when you come home after a meal out *and* you've been able to eat low-GI, lower-fat most of the time. Not only will you feel better, but you should also keep on losing weight – if you've listened to your body correctly.

Meals eaten out are usually much larger than those you'd eat at home. This means that you have, in fact, eaten the quantity of food in one restaurant meal that you would normally eat in two meals at home. At this point, the *art of compensation* is vital for continued weight loss, even when you're faced with a week in which you eat out more than once. Naturally, blood glucose levels will remain higher for much longer, so you probably won't register any hunger by the time the next meal comes around. As we mentioned before, drinking lots of water (or sugar-free cooldrinks, or rooibos tea, low-caffeine tea or decaffeinated coffee with low-fat or skimmed milk and sweetener or little/no sugar) will also help digestion and prevent dehydration after such a concentrated influx of nutrients from a single big meal. Fresh fruit as a "mini-meal" later on may be a sensible choice, but certainly not another full meal. The snacks section (page 164) has plenty of ideas for small snacks.

Here are some tips to help you choose when you're eating out.

Starters
- By far the best way to start a meal is with a salad, especially a French salad, consisting only of salad vegetables. Add an exotic

low-oil dressing or, if that's not possible, ask for the dressing on the side and sprinkle no more than 5 ml (1 t) of dressing over the salad. This salad isn't only a low-fat, low-GI starter, it's also packed with vitamins and minerals that are desperately lacking in the meals we eat in restaurants. As mentioned before, vegetables are also the most filling foods, so the salad starter should help prevent overeating. Beware of Greek salad, however, which can be a fat trap because it contains high-fat olives, medium-fat feta cheese and oily salad dressing. Order half a portion or share with somebody.

◆ Vegetable-based starters are always a good way to begin a meal, provided they're not creamed or crumbed and deep-fat fried. Always choose grilled or baked instead of deep-fat fried dishes.

◆ Asparagus spears with a little low-oil vinaigrette, if available (not with mayonnaise, melted butter or hollandaise sauce).

◆ Grilled mushrooms with lower-fat cheese such as mozzarella.

◆ Grilled mushroom kebab (ask that less, or no, butter or oil be used)

◆ A small portion of smoked salmon.

◆ Fruit skewers are also fun and tasty on a hot summer's night (preferably including lower-GI fruits).

◆ Lean Parma ham with melon balls (even though the melon is high GI, you should be able to balance it out with low-GI vegetables and a low-GI starch with your main meal; see below for ideas).

◆ Grilled calamari (no sauce).

◆ Eat lots of the vegetable snacks at cocktail parties: cucumber and celery sticks, tomatoes, lettuce, asparagus, etc. Decline higher-GI carrots and avoid the high-fat dips and pâtés usually served with them.

◆ Adding a fruit (not melon) or low-GI fruit juice to any meal will also reduce the GI of the meal.

Soups

◆ Choose vegetable-based soups such as minestrone, which has the bonus of containing small white beans ... definitely low GI and lower fat.

◆ Clear broths are also low in fat, and very low in kilojoules, provided that they don't have a layer of fat rings (visible fat layer on the soup) or croutons on top.

◆ Chilled gazpacho is also a good low-fat, low-GI choice.

◆ Chilled cucumber soup or vichyssoise may contain a lot of

cream. Before ordering, make sure the soup was made using low-fat plain yoghurt instead.

◆ Be very wary of creamed soups such as mushroom or butternut soup; they're usually very high in fat and also generally thickened with high-GI flour or cornflour.

◆ Tomato soup, onion soup, bean soup and split pea soup are all good choices.

Main courses

◆ Red meat, chicken and fish choices should always be lean cuts, prepared without added fats. This is quite difficult to achieve in a restaurant, where even "grilled" items are usually smothered in oil or butter during cooking. This is especially true for chicken and fish, as they dry out during cooking, and nobody wants to be served a dried-out chunk of protein. You have to be quite firm and insist you want your meat, fish or chicken to be served dry.

◆ The best red meat choice is a ladies' portion of grilled, trimmed rump or fillet steak, for both men and women. (Remember that trimmed rump contains less fat than trimmed fillet.) Men may eat the whole portion, but a woman should preferably cut off the portion size according to the size of the palm of her hand (see page 117), and take the rest home in a "doggy bag" to be enjoyed on a sandwich the next day. If you listen to your body correctly, you won't be able to finish all your food anyway and would want to take a "doggy bag" home.

◆ It's often better to order deep-fried fish and chicken in batter. Yes, you read correctly! The trick is to eat only the fish or chicken *inside* the batter and to leave the oil-soaked batter on the plate. (Pour water on it if you get tempted to eat it; that will quickly put you off it completely!)

◆ Beware of additional sauces such as cheese sauce which are laden with saturated fat, and may be high GI too if they're thickened with cornflour. Rather choose monkey gland, barbeque, or sweet and sour sauce. Sprinkle a few teaspoons of the sauce over your food, don't drown it in sauce. Remember to ask for the sauce separately, otherwise your food will arrive already drowned in sauce.

◆ Chicken with fillings can be fat traps, e.g. Chicken Kiev which is filled with garlic butter. Rather opt for grilled chicken breasts with a little exotic sauce on the side to tantalise your taste buds. Remember to ask the waiter to have the skin of the chicken removed before grilling!

◆ Chicken kebabs are also a good, lean and tasty choice, as they're usually made from the skinned white meat of chicken.

◆ Seafood as a whole is relatively lean; it's the sauce accompaniments or the preparation method that make for high-fat dishes. Once again, ask for a ladies' portion, as all seafood is high in cholesterol, even when it's grilled.

◆ Calamari rings are usually deep-fat fried and served with tartare sauce, which is made from full-fat mayonnaise. It can, however, also be served grilled or as "steaks" which would be the better choice.

◆ Prawns and crayfish are, in themselves, good lean protein sources. Ask for the sauce to be served separately and just drizzle it over instead of drowning the seafood in sauce.

◆ Be very careful when choosing vegetarian items off a restaurant menu. Most vegetarian dishes are very high in fat as a lot of oil, margarine and cheese are used in their preparation. The fats may be in the pastry of vegetarian pies or quiches, or in the full-cream cheese that generally predominates in these dishes. Cream is often also added.

◆ Pasta dishes can be very deceiving. Choose a sauce that's not made with cream, but based on tomato and herbs, e.g. pasta with a Napoletana sauce or spaghetti bolognaise. If you don't like tomato-based sauces, choose a cream-based sauce, but ask for a half portion of sauce with a double portion of pasta. If you can also add a few cooked vegetables to your plate of food, so much the better. Just make sure they're not drowned in cream, butter and/or sugar.

◆ Add lots of vegetables to your meal. Watch out for glazed vegetables though, as they're high in fat, and should therefore be avoided. The same holds true for creamed vegetables.

◆ Ask for baked beans and add 125 ml ($^1/_2$ C) to your plate as a side dish or, better still, pre-empt the high-GI meal. Decant half a tin of baked beans, lentils or three-bean salad into a plastic container with a tight-fitting lid at home, take it with you and add it to your meal at the social occasion.

◆ Alternatively, you can offer to provide a salad for the social occasion and bring a salad containing beans or other low-GI ingredients, thereby ensuring that the GI of your meal will be reduced. Of course, this doesn't apply when you're going to a restaurant.

◆ Pizzas: Choose lean toppings with lots of vegetables. Good-quality pizzas should be made with lower-fat mozzarella cheese. Beware of added garlic in oil; it shoots the fat content through the roof! Because of the cheese baked on the high-GI pizza base and the presence of low-GI vegetables, the overall GI of pizza is generally intermediate, which is quite acceptable, especially if you combine it with three-bean salad, another low-GI salad or a small low-GI fruit juice. You can also ask for less cheese to reduce the fat content slightly, as some pizzerias use far too much cheese anyway.

◆ Hamburgers need to be "doctored" to reduce the GI and the fat content. Drop the chips and opt for the salad bar instead. Choose salads with no dressings or low-oil dressings, and look for the bean salad. Ask the waiter or owner whether it contains oil, however, otherwise you could find you have too generous a portion! Eat half the roll only and watch out for high-fat sauces.

Bread and starches

◆ Most rolls and breads served with meals in restaurants are high GI and should be avoided. Only dense, heavy breads, spread with the minimum of butter or margarine, may be eaten. If they're not available, at least try some combining, for example, have low-GI bean salad with the hamburger or a small apple juice, etc.

◆ Remember to add a low-GI starch to your meat dish. Ask for baby potatoes (with skin) instead of a baked potato or chips, which are high GI and/or high fat. Basmati rice is also available in most restaurants today, and some even serve sweet potatoes. Pasta's also a popular menu item, so don't be shy to ask for pasta as your starch, even if your dish isn't normally served with it.

◆ Rice: The GI value of most South African rice has not yet been determined, but most restaurants use loose rice, which usually has a lower GI value. Most of our clients who prefer rice with their restaurant meal, find their blood glucose levels are fine the next morning. So choose rice as your starch, rather than high-GI potatoes, mash or chips.

Dessert

Unfortunately, most desserts are both high GI and high in fat. A dessert that's fruit- or dairy-based, without cream, is acceptable, however. The list below contains the better choices; they're lower GI, but strictly speaking not lower fat. It would be best if you didn't have dessert at all, but if you have to eat it, at least choose one of the following lower-GI options (or share one of these options with someone):

◆ Crème caramel
◆ Crème brûlée
◆ Blancmange
◆ Cheesecake (preferably low-fat)
◆ Fruit salad and ice cream (preferably low-fat ice cream)
◆ Custard (preferably low-fat)
◆ Fruit jelly whip
◆ Milktart
◆ Apple pudding/cake/tart/crumble (try to leave some of the pastry and eat more of the filling)
◆ Apple strudel
◆ Low-fat yoghurt as the dessert will lower the GI of any meal.

Next time you go out for a meal, read through this section again before you leave and choose the three tips that apply best in the current situation, then try to implement them. See how good you'll feel when you've eaten out, enjoyed yourself and don't have to feel guilty about having eaten the wrong foods.

The best and easiest, of course, would be if restaurants or take-away places served a lower-fat, lower-GI menu as an alternative to the standard menu. A few restaurants do, by serving a GIFSA-endorsed menu that's a lower-fat, lower-GI version of their standard menu, and that was compiled for them by one of the GIFSA dieticians. Look out for the GIFSA endorsement on restaurant menus, as the registered dietician who compiled it has already done the thinking for you! Any of the options on a GIFSA-endorsed menu would be safe on a slimming diet, for those with diabetes, high blood cholesterol levels and high blood pressure, among other conditions, but just as tasty.

If you'd like your favourite restaurant, coffee shop or take-away to serve a GIFSA-endorsed menu, ask them to contact GIFSA at dellas@mweb.co.za.

Meals for a week

Note: See pages 191 – 214 for the recipes of dishes with an asterisk (*).

Breakfast

Continental summer breakfast

Place some chopped low-GI fresh fruit or Fruit salad* in a large pudding bowl. Top with low-fat fruit yoghurt and sprinkle with some low-GI muesli for added crunch.

Follow this with a low-GI muffin* with low-GI jam and grated low-fat cheese.

Add a large glass of water or unsweetened iced tea.

Specifics:

- 125 ml ($^1/_2$ C) low-GI Fruit salad* (about 120 g) *or* 1 low-GI fruit, grated or finely chopped
- 1 small tub, *or* 100 ml, *or* $^1/_2$ x 175 ml tub, *or* 2 heaped dessert-spoons (about 80 ml) out of a large container of low-fat, sweetened fruit yoghurt
- 1 heaped dessertspoon (about 30-40 ml) low-GI muesli (e.g. Fine Form, *or* one of Nature's Source low-GI mueslis, *or* one of the mueslis from *Eating for Sustained Energy*, pages 28, 29, 34)
- 1 low-GI muffin*
- 5 ml (1 tsp) low-GI jam, e.g. Fine Form jam
- $^1/_2$ "matchbox" (15 g) grated low-fat cheese, e.g. Lichten Blanc or Woolworths' low-fat Cheddar or Gouda
- 1 large glass water or unsweetened iced tea

Winter breakfast

Start with orange segments or $^1/_2$ grapefruit

Follow with low-GI oats porridge cooked with half water and half skimmed milk, sweetened with raw honey

End off with Cape seed loaf and avocado, topped with shaved ham or chicken and seasoned with black pepper

Tea or coffee and low-fat/skimmed milk

Specifics:

- 1 orange, cut into segments, or $^1/_2$ grapefruit

- 65 ml ($^1/_4$ cup) or 1 heaped dessertspoon (about 40 ml) raw low-GI oats porridge (e.g. Bokomo, Woolworths oats) cooked with 125 ml ($^1/_2$ C) skimmed milk and water
- 5 ml (1 level t) raw honey
- 1 thin slice Cape seed loaf
- 1 – 2 thin slices avocado (5 mm thick)
- 1 – 2 paper-thin slices (15 g) of shaved ham or chicken
- Tea or decaffeinated coffee with low-fat or skimmed milk and a little sugar or sweetener if desired

Breakfast treat
Start with low-GI Fruit salad* and top it with fat-free fruit yoghurt.
Then have two low-GI crumpets*.
Spread the first with low-GI jam and a little whipped cream
Add chopped lean bacon to the second crumpet
Finish off with decaffeinated cappuccino made with
skimmed milk froth.

Specifics:
- 125 ml ($^1/_2$ C) low-GI Fruit salad*
- 125 ml ($^1/_2$ C) fat-free fruit yoghurt (e.g. Pick 'n Pay Choice, Clover Danone or Woolworths)
- Two low-GI crumpets*
- 5 ml (1 level t) low-GI jam (e.g. Fine Form)
- 10 ml (1 heaped t) whipped cream
- 1 – 2 rashers lean bacon, fat removed before cooking, then grilled or fake-fried and chopped (see Fake-frying [page 132])
- Decaffeinated cappuccino made with 125 ml ($^1/_2$ C) skimmed milk froth

Health breakfast on the run
Quickly whip together a fruit whip made up of:
plain yoghurt, low-GI fruits,
chopped nuts and raw honey

Specifics:
- 175 ml tub, *or* $^1/_3$ of a 500 ml tub of low-fat/fat-free plain yoghurt
- 2 low-GI fruits (e.g. apple, pear, orange, peach, kiwifruit, plums, apricots) *or*

◆ 1 low-GI and 1 intermediate-GI fruit (e.g. 1 small banana, *or* 1 small mango *or* a slice of pawpaw)
◆ A small portion of nuts (e.g. 10 pecan halves [chopped], *or* 20 peanuts, *or* 5 almonds, *or* 10 cashews)
◆ 5 ml (1 level t) raw honey or soft brown sugar

Quick breakfast
Start your day with some fruit.
Add an instant low-GI cereal or a mixture of two or three of them with low-fat or skimmed milk.
Finish off with a big glass of water.
Specifics:
◆ 1 slice pawpaw with lemon juice to reduce the GI slightly
◆ 125 ml – 250 ml ($^1/_2$ – 1 C) low-GI cereal (e.g. Wholewheat Pronutro [Original or Applebake]; Fine Form muesli; Nature's Source low-GI muesli; low-GI muesli recipes in *Eating for Sustained Energy* [pages 28, 30, 34]; Bokomo Maximize; Kellogg's High Fibre Bran; Jungle Oat Bran)
◆ 125 ml – 250 ml ($^1/_2$ – 1 C) skimmed or low-fat milk
◆ Remember your big glass of water!

Farmstyle breakfast
Start off with a small glass of freshly squeezed low-GI fruit juice.
Then put together a delicious cooked breakfast of egg and lean bacon, grilled tomato, mushroom and onion, baked beans and low-GI toast.
Finish off this delicious breakfast with a steaming cup of tea or decaffeinated coffee with low-fat or fat-free milk.
Specifics:
◆ One wineglass of freshly squeezed low-GI fruit juice (see GI list on page 222.)
◆ First fake-fry (see page 132) one rasher of lean bacon, fat removed (e.g. Like it Lean) with the onion. Remove to a serving plate.
◆ Add the egg and cook. Remove to a serving plate.
◆ Lastly, add the mushrooms and tomato and cook until done.
◆ Heat 125 ml ($^1/_2$ C) or $^1/_2$ small tin (200 g) baked beans.

◆ Serve the cooked breakfast with 1 thin slice of seed loaf or rye bread (no margarine or butter).

◆ End the meal with tea or decaffeinated coffee with low-fat or skimmed milk and a little sugar or sweetener if desired.

Delicious low-GI, lower-fat lunches

Open chicken mayo sandwich with three-bean salad and mineral water

Specifics:

◆ 125 ml ($^1/_2$ C) three-bean salad*, or readymade low-oil three-bean salad

◆ 1 slice brown bread (the low-GI beans in the salad will cancel the effect of the high-GI brown bread).

◆ Put on the bread: 1 tomato, sliced, plus 1 baby cucumber, sliced

◆ Mix together:
10 ml (1 heaped t) low-fat mayonnaise
2 ml ($^1/_2$ t) whole-grain mustard
$^1/_2$ chicken breast, shredded

◆ Pile the chicken mayo onto the slice of bread and serve with the salad.

◆ 1 glass mineral water.

Pasta and chicken salad for 4

Specifics:

◆ Combine:
500 ml (2 C) cooked pasta, *or* pearled wheat, *or* pearled barley
410 g tin baked beans in tomato sauce
4 drumsticks, *or* 2 thighs of lean chicken, *or* 4 lean Viennas (e.g. Like it Lean), *or* 180 g tin tuna in brine
$^1/_2$ tomato, chopped
$^1/_2$ green and $^1/_2$ red pepper
20 ml (1 heaped T) lite or low-fat mayonnaise
2 heaped dessertspoons (about 80 ml) low-fat plain yoghurt
10 ml (1 heaped t) fruity chutney
freshly ground black pepper

◆ Place one quarter of the pasta and protein mixture on washed lettuce leaves on four individual plates and enjoy!

Make the whole recipe for *four* people. It's so delicious, you'll want to have it again and again. This also makes a wonderful packed lunch. Chill and take to work in an airtight container, then enjoy this summertime treat for lunch.

More than just a sandwich

Specifics:

◆ Take 2 slices of seed loaf, wheat-free rye bread or pumpernickel and top the first slice with a mixture made up of:
$^1/_4$ tub (50-60 g) low-fat or fat-free cottage cheese
5 ml (1 level t) raw honey
some whole-grain mustard
5 ml (1 t) soya sauce
5 ml (1 t) chopped chives
5 ml (1 level t) sesame seeds
Spread on the slice of bread and top with tomato slices.

◆ Cover the second slice with:
$^1/_4$ small or $^1/_8$ medium avocado
add 1 – 2 slices of shaved chicken or ham
add a few slivers of Mediterranean cocktail peppadews.

◆ Place both open sandwiches on a fancy dinner plate, decorate with a variety of lettuce leaves and enjoy a gourmet meal.

◆ To finish off, enjoy a glass of fruity rooibos tea: Add 125 ml ($^1/_2$ C) low-GI fruit juice, e.g. Ceres Secrets of the Valley juice, to cold rooibos tea.

The low-GI cracker quintet

Specifics:

◆ Take 5 low-GI crackers and top with any *one* of the following per cracker:

◆ 2 mm slice of Brie cheese (enough to cover the cracker) and freshly ground black pepper

◆ Low-fat or fat-free cottage cheese rosettes with slivers of smoked salmon

◆ 2 – 3 paper-thin slices of mozzarella cheese interleaved with tomato slices marinated in balsamic vinegar

◆ Low-fat or fat-free cottage cheese, chopped peppadews and pickled cucumber

◆ 5 ml (1 t) grated biltong, sprinkled on either cottage cheese or mashed avocado
◆ A few thin apple and cheese slices, alternating on the cracker
◆ 5 ml (1 t) grated medium-fat cheese (e.g. In Shape or Elite fat-reduced cheddar) with sun-dried tomatoes
◆ Brinjal pâté*

Toasted cheese with a difference
Specifics:
◆ Take 1 – 2 slices of low-GI bread and top with the following:
Lettuce, finely shredded
Tomato, chopped
Cucumber, chopped
1 "matchbox" (30 g) grated mozzarella cheese on top
◆ Microwave on high for 1 minute and enjoy!

Filled bread roll
Specifics:
Take one of your favourite high-GI bread rolls, *or* pita bread, *or* low-fat Taco shell and fill with the following:
◆ 125 ml – 250 ml ($^1/_2$ – 1 C) canned butter beans or any other beans you have in stock (it's imperative to use beans as your protein with a bread roll, white or brown, in order to compensate for the high-GI roll)
◆ Chopped veggies of your choice, e.g. lettuce or cabbage, cucumber, gherkins, tomato, mushrooms, peppadews, green or red peppers, etc.
◆ Low-fat dressing: 20 ml (1 heaped T) low-fat mayonnaise mixed with a little skimmed milk
◆ Sweet basil and black pepper to taste

Suppers
Pasta 'n sauce
Specifics:
◆ Cook your favourite pasta shapes in lightly salted water, then add one of the low-fat pasta sauces* (tomato, vegetable or mushroom) in the recipe section.

- Add a mixed vegetable salad to balance the meal.
- For those needing more protein, add 1 round or stick of Feta cheese to the salad, or grate 1 "matchbox" (30 g) of low- or medium-fat cheese over the pasta and sauce, *or* double your portion of the sauce.

Grilled chicken breast combo

For a really delicious and snappy meal, try this easy supper:
Specifics:
- Brush 1 skinned chicken breast or thigh fillet (per person) with a mixture of:
  sweet chilli sauce, soy sauce and chopped fresh coriander
  Cook on a braai (barbecue) or grill.
- Add a tossed salad (not carrot or beetroot)
- Serve with roast sweet potato & butternut*

Fish burgers

Load up on Omega-3 essential fatty acids by having these fish burgers once a week.
Specifics:
- Make up a fish burger using the following:
  1 fish burger patty*
  1 small bread roll, preferably brown/wholewheat for the fibre
  20 ml (1 heaped T) low-fat or lite mayonnaise
  Lettuce, bean sprouts
  Tomato sauce
  1 thin slice pineapple
- Finish off the meal with 125 ml ($^1/_2$ C) low-GI fresh fruit salad*, since both the bread roll and the pineapple have higher GI values.
- Top with vanilla sauce made from a little plain low-fat or fat-free yoghurt, a little sugar to taste and a few drops of vanilla essence.

Quick pork medallions with mushroom sauce

Specifics:
- Thickly slice a pork fillet into 3 cm thick medallions (2 medallions per person) and fake-fry (see page 132)
- Serve with 65 ml ($^1/_4$ C) mushroom sauce*, 125 ml ($^1/_2$ C)

basmati rice mixed with 65 ml ($^1/_4$ C) canned or cooked lentils, and cooked broccoli/cauliflower and sugarsnap peas, or any other vegetables.

Soup supper

Specifics:

♦ Vegetable Soup* (350 ml)
♦ Grilled seed loaf cheezie*, *or* 1 portion Apple crumble* and 65 ml ($^1/_4$ C) custard*

Snacks

It's very important to make sure that you eat low-GI, lower-fat snacks when you need to eat between meals. Remember that a high-GI snack will only make you hungrier within the hour, and you'll want to eat again and again. See explanation of how the Glycemic Index works on page 79.

Here are some low-GI, lower-fat snacks that will help you through your *snack attack*. But remember that you should preferably eat only three meals a day and you might have to compensate for the snack at your next meal. That's why we thought it best to differentiate between "meal snacks" and "snack snacks".

Meal snacks

These are more substantial snacks, which are actually very similar in composition to a light meal. If you have one of these meal snacks with your morning or afternoon tea or coffee, you actually don't need the full meal at lunch or supper that follows.

This is where you learn to *compensate*. Having had a "meal snack", you'll only need a snack at the next meal instead of a full meal, as you won't really be hungry enough to eat a full meal.

Any one of the "snack snacks", or a salad consisting mainly of vegetables and a little protein, would be suitable.

Carrot cake with tea or coffee

Specifics:

♦ 1 portion Carrot cake* ($^1/_{12}$ of the cake) with tea, preferably rooibos or low-caffeine tea, or decaffeinated coffee with low-fat/fat-free milk and a little sugar or sweetener if desired.

◆ Remember that caffeine can raise blood pressure, as well as blood cholesterol and blood glucose levels, which can lead to high blood glucose in diabetics and *reactive* hypoglycaemia in healthy individuals, but especially in those suffering from hypoglycaemia. This is one of the reasons we recommend that you limit your intake of ordinary coffee to one cup a day.

Low-fat, low-GI muffin* with tea or coffee
Specifics:

◆ 1 low-fat, low-GI muffin* with a cup of rooibos tea, low-caffeine tea or decaffeinated coffee with low-fat/fat-free milk and a little sugar or sweetener if desired. Try to have the muffin without a spread, jam, cheese or anything else.

◆ It's easier to bake a whole batch of muffins and freeze them until needed. To defrost, microwave on high for 20 seconds per muffin.

Low-GI cracker duo or trio
Specifics:

◆ 2 – 3 low-GI crackers with any one of the listed toppings (see Lunches, page 160) per cracker

◆ A big glass of water.

"Snack snacks"
The fresh fruit "in-betweener"
Always keep fresh fruit in the vegetable drawer of your fridge, so that the juiciest, freshest fruit is available to you at any time of day. A single piece of fruit is still the best-packaged, healthiest and best low-GI, low-fat snack around.
Specifics:

◆ Choose 1 to 2 pieces of low-GI fresh fruit as the perfect in-between munchie.

◆ See fruits in the GI list at the back of this book (page 221).

Dried fruit medley

Specifics:
- Choose only *two* of the following:
  4 dried apricot halves
  2 – 3 dried apple rings
  2 dried peach halves
  2 dried prunes
- Add a generous glass of water.

Emergency snack

Specifics:
- 200 ml low-fat sweetened drinking yoghurt, any flavour, any brand.
- Remember that all yoghurt, sweetened and unsweetened, has a low-GI value.

Yoghurt to the rescue

Specifics:
- 1 small tub (100 ml) low-fat sweetened fruit yoghurt *or*
- $^1/_2$ tub 175 ml low-fat sweetened fruit yoghurt, *or*
- 1 small tub (125 ml) fat-free, fructose-sweetened fruit yoghurt, *or*
- 1 small tub (175 ml) fat-free, sugar-free fruit yoghurt, any flavour, *or*
- 1 small tub (175 ml) plain low-fat or fat-free yoghurt, flavoured with vanilla, strawberry or other essence of your choice and sweetener or 5 ml (1 t) sugar or raw honey.

Stewed fruit and custard

Specifics:
- Choose *one* of the following stewed fruit portions:
  4 dried apricot halves
  2 – 3 dried apple rings
  2 dried peach halves
  2 dried prunes
- Add 2 heaped dessertspoons (about 80ml) of low-fat custard.

Section 3

Activity

Chapter 7

How active are you?

Activity questionnaire

Are you active enough?

Read each question carefully and then choose the answer (A to E) that you agree with *most:*

A – don't agree at all
B – don't agree totally
C – don't always agree
D – agree mostly
E – agree 100%

If you choose A you agree least with the statement, and if you choose E you agree completely. For each question, circle the number under the headings A to E, then add up the numbers at the end of the questionnaire to get your score.

		Agree the least				Agree the most
		A	B	C	D	E
1.	I have never followed an exercise programme	5	4	3	2	1
2.	I really dislike exercise	5	4	3	2	1
3.	How many times in a week do you exercise?	1	2	3	4	5
4.	When I exercise I usually: go to the gym, run, cycle, go for a brisk walk, dance, swim, play underwater hockey, train for a triathlon or do contact sport	1	2	3	4	5
5.	I sit at a desk at work	5	4	3	2	1
6.	I quickly get out of breath when I do anything physical	5	4	3	4	5
7.	Over weekends I run/cycle a long distance, exercise for more than an hour in the gym, dance for more than an hour or take part in sport, e.g. tennis, hockey, rugby, etc.	1	2	3	4	5
8.	In my free time I usually read, watch TV, play computer games, sew, knit or go to the movies	5	4	3	2	1
9.	In my free time I usually play action cricket, roller blade, go for a brisk walk, work in the garden, do woodwork or work on my motorbike or motorcar	1	2	3	4	5
10.	I don't have time to exercise	5	4	3	2	1

How did you score?

Note: Double your score to get a percentage (%).

0 – 40%

This score indicates that you're basically inactive and probably unfit as well. To lose weight you'll have to lead a more active lifestyle, and start a regular exercise programme. By doing this, you'll not only begin to lose weight, you'll also decrease your risk of contracting lifestyle diseases such as diabetes, insulin resistance, heart disease, gout, high blood pressure, etc.

41 – 70%

With a score of over 40, you can consider yourself a reasonably active person. Your lifestyle involves a good dose of physical activity, or you follow a regular exercise programme, or both. You should lose weight successfully on a slimming diet, and be able to maintain your weight on a maintenance plan. If you eat healthily and keep up this level of exercise, you won't increase your risk for lifestyle diseases.

70%+

A score of more than 70 indicates that you're probably a serious athlete, or at least do more exercise than the average active person. Being overweight shouldn't be one of your concerns, unless you consume too much fat, take in too much energy (kilojoules), or eat the wrong kind of carbohydrates, at the wrong time. Your level of fitness will help to protect you against the lifestyle diseases, provided that you follow a healthy diet.

Chapter 8

The importance of exercise

The disadvantages of not exercising

1. Eating less, without increasing activity, hampers weight loss

Many of our clients tell us they'd rather go hungry than exercise. It seems a pity that people are so "allergic" to exercise, and would do anything rather than exercise. Eating less can have a negative connotation, whereas doing exercise is positive.

Some people also like to point out that our forefathers ate almost anything they wanted to, and didn't suffer from our modern lifestyle diseases, such as high cholesterol levels, diabetes, etc. In fact, many of them reached old age. What most people forget, however, is that medical science was not as advanced in the diagnosis of disease at that time, and our forefathers were much more active than we are today. They grew their own vegetables, milked the cows and made cheese and butter from the milk, and so on. They also walked to work, used a bicycle or rode to work on a horse.

In stark contrast, most of us drive to work, use the escalator or elevator to get to the office, sit in front of a computer or at a desk all day, then drive home again at night. In other words, we live a life completely devoid of any physical activity. Not many people would consider walking to visit a friend or to go shopping; the car is used every single time we want to go anywhere.

Eating less, without exercise, results in lean body mass loss (muscle loss), and a reduction in the basal metabolic rate (BMR). It's easier for the body to use protein (muscle) for energy than to use fat stores. This is especially true when energy intake is drastically reduced to less than 4 200 kilojoules (1 000 calories) a day, as is the case with most fad diets. As explained in the discussion on very low kilojoule diets (page 61), when your energy intake is too low, your body thinks it's under threat and stores fat to ensure you'll survive the perceived food shortage. This loss of body protein (muscle) for energy has the effect of lowering your basal metabolic rate even more, as it's determined by your lean body mass. In addition, research has shown that the weight loss promised by very low kilojoule diets is only 50% fat loss – the rest is loss of precious lean body mass and water. Most of these diets also advise against exercise, which is just as well, as you wouldn't have the energy to exercise!

2. The natural decline in metabolic rate and muscle tone with age is aggravated by inactivity

It's a known fact that the metabolic rate (the speed at which your body burns the food you eat to get energy) slows down with age – about 2% every ten years. This may not sound like a lot, but if you were to eat an extra 88 kilojoules a day (more or less, half a biscuit), you'd gain 10 kg in ten years. So a woman with a basal metabolic rate (BMR) of 6 300 kJ a day needs to reduce her daily intake by 126 kJ every ten years to maintain her weight at what it was when she was 25. This is what we'd all have to do, if we didn't exercise. If we didn't, we could gain 10 kg every ten years.

Age also erodes muscle tone, resulting in "jodhpur thighs" in women and a large stomach in men. And to add insult to injury, loss of muscle tone further reduces the metabolic rate. Exercise is one of the few ways we have to keep our metabolic rate up and help to keep muscle tone.

3. Lack of exercise increases your risk for insulin resistance, metabolic syndrome (Syndrome X) and other lifestyle diseases

The metabolic syndrome or Syndrome X is characterised by over-weight or obesity, hyperinsulinaemia, insulin resistance, glucose intolerance (low blood sugar or diabetes), high cholesterol levels, high blood pressure, hyperlipidaemia, chronic candida infections and, very often, polycystic ovarian syndrome (PCOS). Most over-weight or obese people have high insulin levels and are insulin resistant. Insulin resistance happens when the pancreas pours out huge quantities of insulin and literally drowns body cells in insulin so that they forget to react properly. Remember, insulin is the hor-mone that helps to push glucose into the cells for energy, and if the cells aren't receiving the energy and the glucose stays in the blood-stream, your body will make more insulin in an attempt to reduce blood glucose levels. Again the cells are drowned and cannot react properly, and the vicious cycle continues. The only way to stop this is to reduce the high insulin levels (hyperinsulinaemia), so that the insulin resistance also disappears.

Anything that reduces hyperinsulinaemia and insulin resistance will enhance insulin sensitivity and induce weight loss, reduce cho-lesterol levels, reduce blood pressure and lipid (blood fat) levels, give better blood sugar control, combat chronic candida infections and PCOS. Exercise has the ability to counteract both high insulin levels and insulin resistance. And exercise combined with a low GI, lower fat diet can reduce insulin resistance and high insulin levels. (To recap on how eating low-GI and lower-fat foods can prevent hyper-insulinaemia and insulin resistance, see page 85).

Apart from the fact that inactivity aggravates hyperinsulinaemia and insulin resistance, inactive people usually suffer from higher cholesterol and lipid levels, high blood pressure, and blood glucose control problems. This means they're at risk for all the lifestyle dis-eases. By increasing their activity levels, they reduce this risk. For all the above reasons, and many more, you need to make exercise your best friend.

4. Inactive people tend to eat more

Remember the discussion in Section 1 on how physical activities can distract you from thinking about food and eating? Not only do physical activities keep your mind off food and eating, but while doing the activity, you're also using up more energy.

The saying, "the devil makes work for idle hands" is particularly relevant when it comes to exercise. You'd have to agree that it's easier to snack on chips, dried wors, biltong and other high-fat snacks while watching sport on TV, than if you were out jogging, or playing tennis or cricket. Knowing that you're going to compete in a sports event, you'd eat only a small meal at least an hour before the event, so that you don't feel nauseous or uncomfortable during the event. Physical activity can also be an appetite suppressant, so much so that some people aren't hungry after they've exercised. In contrast, being inactive tends to lead to eating, and this can be prevented by getting involved in some form of physical activity.

The human body needs a certain amount of physical activity to ensure that the hunger and satiety signals work properly. Inactive people usually have a bigger appetite and consequently tend to eat more and gain weight easily, quite apart from the fact that they also have a slower metabolism.

5. Inactivity results in being unfit

Fitness can be lost in a very short space of time, once you stop exercising. This can result in shortness of breath, sleeplessness, muscle cramps, and even constipation.

The advantages of regular exercise

Exercise has so many benefits that, once you've read this section, you'll wonder why you haven't been exercising all your life!

1. Regular exercise allows you to eat more, even on a slimming diet, because you burn more energy

When you're active and exercise regularly, you'll be able to eat more and still lose weight, so people who'd rather eat less than exercise are actually shooting themselves in the foot. Your basal metabolic rate (BMR) can be calculated by any dietician and then the energy required for your activities is added on to get to your energy require-ments for the day. The dietician will then be able to work out what your energy requirements should be per day, for you to lose weight. Generally, you will need to eat 4 200 kJ less per day to lose 1 kg body fat a week. So the middle-aged woman mentioned earlier (page 173) would have to consume only 2 100 kJ a day in order to lose 1 kg a week! No dietician would put anyone on a diet that contains less than 4 200 kJ a day, however, as this would slow down the metabolism. So this woman will have to be satisfied with a 500 g loss a week. Should she be exercising regularly, however, her BMR would increase to be-tween 7 560 kJ and 8 400 kJ a day, which means she would lose 1 kg a week, and reach her goal weight without becoming despondent.

2. Regular exercise can increase your BMR (basal metabolic rate)

Many people tend to embrace all sorts of solutions that don't require any physical effort, in an attempt to increase their metabolism (caf-feine, chromium, amino acids, ginseng, etc.). To date, no miracle cure has been discovered that can enhance the rate at which your body burns fat. The only way to increase your BMR, without harm-ing your body, is to increase your physical activity. The oldest, and still the most effective, way to lose weight is to combine a balanced diet with exercise. By following the low-GI, lower-fat diet and em-bracing an exercise programme, you can be sure you'll lose body fat, not precious lean body mass.

How exercise increases your metabolic rate:

◆ *While doing exercise, you burn kilojoules.* The table on page 186 shows how many kilojoules are used for various activities. Being active burns up at least 315 kJ per half hour whereas sitting still, even if you're working at a computer, only uses up 168 kJ – 210 kJ. Imagine how little you need while lying down!

◆ *Exercising is like compound interest.* If you run a standard marathon for two to three hours, your body will burn 1 260 kJ – 1 890 kJ every half hour, and your BMR (the rate at which your body burns energy) will be increased for the rest of the day, sometimes even for a few days after the event. For example, a not-so-active middle-aged woman will have a BMR of 6 300 kJ a day. If she takes up jogging, and eventually runs for an hour every day, she can increase her BMR to 7 560 kJ a day. On a day when she runs two to three hours, her BMR will be higher than 7 560 kJ and it will remain elevated for a few days afterwards.

◆ Regular exercise *helps to maintain muscle tone*, especially with resistance exercise, such as weight training, Callanetics, Pilates, etc. Your BMR is, to a certain extent, determined by muscle tone, so keeping your muscles toned would go a long way towards keeping your BMR up, rather than having it decrease over the years as it normally would.

3. Physical activity improves insulin sensitivity and decreases the risk for insulin resistance, obesity, diabetes and other lifestyle diseases

Physical activity improves insulin sensitivity in the following manner. Every cell in your body has a number of insulin receptors, or "glucose catchers". If you're one of those unlucky people who have only one or two insulin receptors on each cell surface, your body cells will have difficulty taking glucose from the bloodstream, and you'll be more prone to developing insulin resistance than someone who has three or four insulin receptors on each cell surface. The number of insulin receptors can, however, be increased by exercising and consuming a low-GI, lower-fat, high-fibre diet. This means that your body's ability to take glucose from the bloodstream, with the help of insulin, will be improved. Because of the reduction in hyperinsulinaemia and insulin resistance, weight loss will become easier.

As mentioned before, most overweight people suffer from insulin resistance. By doing just one intense bout of exercise a week, they can reduce their risk of developing diabetes by as much as 33%.

The ability to control blood glucose levels diminishes with age, so it becomes very important to remain physically active as we get older. The insulin levels per se don't drop, but insulin sensitivity does. Physical activity can help to stabilise blood glucose levels and body mass in the middle-aged and elderly.

High-intensity exercise, such as aerobics, running and squash, reduces insulin levels and increases glucagon levels in the blood. This in turn increases the production of good prostaglandins that improve blood circulation (by supplying oxygen and nutrients to the cells) and increases the body's ability to burn fat – an ideal situation for weight loss.

Physical activity also increases the level of HDL, or "good" cholesterol (yes, there is such a thing!) which removes the "bad" LDL and VLDL (very low density lipoprotein) cholesterol from the blood. People who have high HDL cholesterol levels are usually more active than those with low levels, and as a result have a much smaller chance of having a heart attack or stroke than their inactive friends.

4. Exercise is a natural appetite suppressant

Even moderate exercise reduces the appetite, although most people believe the opposite to be true. Recent studies have shown that appetite decreases with increased physical activity.

5. Physical activity releases endorphins

During exercise, your body releases hormones called endorphins. They instil a feeling of wellbeing and a zest for life, which makes losing weight a whole lot easier. High levels of endorphins can be addictive, but this kind of addiction is perhaps better than gambling, or alcoholism. The fact that many athletes train year in and year out for marathons is proof of this addiction. Only the high of endorphin release during the Comrades Marathon, for instance, can explain why athletes flock together at the start of the race, when they know full well that they'll suffer for the next few days.

Laughing also releases endorphins, as does eating. It would be counter-productive to get your daily dose of endorphins from eating, so the best way is to get into the habit of exercising every day, and to laugh a lot.

6. You can eat a wider variety of foods when you're active

After exercise, higher-GI foods are recommended to keep blood glucose levels from dropping too much. So, having exercised, you're free to eat any kind of carbohydrate and aren't restricted to eating only low-GI carbohydrates. Without exercise, you're limited to eating only low-GI foods to ensure a steady stream of energy between meals. By eating low GI, you promote weight loss, whereas consumption of high-GI foods, without exercise, would result in tiredness and an increased risk of developing one or more of the lifestyle diseases.

The *general rule* is that everybody should eat lower-fat, low-GI foods when inactive and before exercise. Only after exercise should intermediate- or high-GI foods be consumed. This concept will be discussed in greater depth in the next paragraphs.

Sport nutrition guidelines

When considering an exercise programme or any kind of sport, it's important that you understand how to enhance your performance and endurance, and that you choose something you can do for the rest of your life. From a nutritional perspective, regulating body fuel is all-important. So let us teach you how to optimise your "petrol" levels before, during and after exercise.

Before exercise

Studies over the last 20 years have shown that low-GI carbohydrates, consumed before exercise, have two advantages:
1. They improve the body's fat-burning ability during exercise, as only small quantities of insulin are released before and during the exercise.
2. Endurance is enhanced.

The pre-event meal guideline for prolonged exercise (tennis matches or a marathon, for instance) is *1g of low GI carbohydrates per kg body mass.*

So a woman weighing 50 kg requires 50 g low-GI carbohydrate before running a marathon. This means she could have 375 ml (1½ C) low-GI cooked pasta (durum wheat) or cooled mealiemeal porridge. The pasta could be served with a tomato and onion sauce and the cooled mealiemeal porridge with low-fat milk and sugar, keeping the protein and fat to a minimum.

A comprehensive list of low-GI carbohydrates, in portions of 50 g or 75 g, is available from any dietician who uses the Glycemic Index in the treatment of clients. See GIFSA's website (www.gifoundation. com) for a list of such dieticians.

If you're less serious about your sport, a small low-GI snack, for example an apple, 30 – 60 minutes before exercise will be sufficient.

If, however, you've eaten a meal one to two hours before exercising, you don't require a low-GI snack. If you choose not to have some low-GI food before exercising you may burn more fat, but you'll find it difficult to exercise for very long before fatigue sets in. (See page 163 for more low-GI meal and snack ideas suitable for before exercise.)

During exercise

Researchers working in the field of sport nutrition generally agree that people who consume carbohydrates during a long exercise session perform better, although this depends on the duration and intensity of the exercise.

If you exercise for an hour or less at a time you won't require extra fuel during the exercise session, except for water. (Provided, of course, that you've eaten a low-GI meal or snack beforehand.) This applies especially to those wanting to lose weight.

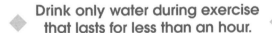

**Drink only water during exercise
that lasts for less than an hour.**

If you exercise for more than an hour and a half at a time (underwater hockey, swimming, long-distance cycling, running, etc.) you will need an additional high-GI carbohydrate during exercise, over and above the low-GI meal or snack before exercise. The following guidelines apply:

◆ 0,5 g high-GI carbohydrate per kg body mass and 250 ml (1 C) water per hour, after 90 minutes' exercise.

◆ For those with diabetes: 0,5g intermediate-GI carbohydrate per kg body mass and 250 ml (1 C) water per hour, after 90 minutes' exercise.

This means that *a sportsman or woman who has diabetes*, or any person with sensitive blood glucose control, should rather drink cooldrinks sweetened with sugar, such as Fanta, or any fruit juice with an intermediate GI, during exercise. (See the GI lists at the back of this book for specific fruit juices that have intermediate GI values.) The drink may be diluted with water. Someone weighing 75 kg, for example, will have to consume 500 ml (2 C) fruit juice or cool-drink every hour to get the required quantity of carbohydrate.

A *healthy sportswoman or -man*, on the other hand, can consume high-GI carbohydrates if they exercise for longer than 90 minutes. A 75 kg man, for instance, would need 500 ml (2 C) of a sports drink every hour during the exercise.

Consuming the carbohydrate with water improves stamina and concentration.

After exercise

It's very important to consume a higher-GI food or drink within 30 – 60 minutes of finishing exercise.

During exercise, glycogen (glucose) stores in the muscle tissues are depleted. Once you stop exercising, your muscles have first priority on any glucose there may be in the blood, in order to replenish glycogen stores. This means that blood glucose levels can drop dramatically after exercise because all the glucose is taken up by the muscles (known as the "sponge effect"). As a result you feel exhausted and may just want to sleep, as you're totally out of fuel and your brain can only function properly when it receives a steady supply of glucose.

To prevent this happening, we recommend that you eat or drink *1 g high-GI carbohydrate per kg body mass 30 – 60 minutes after exercise.*

For those with diabetes: eat or drink 1 g intermediate-GI carbohydrate per kg body mass 30 – 60 minutes after exercise.

If you exercise for less than one hour a day, an intermediate-GI carbohydrate snack (e.g. a banana) should be enough after exercise. If you exercise for less than an hour just before your next meal, you can choose an intermediate-GI starch with your meal, e.g. brown rice, or a sandwich plus a low-GI fruit. Together, the high-GI bread and the low-GI fruit make an intermediate-GI meal.

Anyone who exercises for more than one hour every day should follow these recommendations. So a person weighing 60 kg, for example, needs 500 ml (2 C) high-GI drink, e.g. a sports drink (see GI lists at the back of the book) after his or her exercise of one hour or more. Should this person have diabetes, an intermediate-GI drink is called for, e.g. fruit juice such as grape juice. Subsequent meals or snacks can be lower GI, but the longer you've exercised and the greater the intensity, the longer you can eat high-GI food afterwards. Each person is unique. For this reason it is important to experiment to find out what works for you. If you need help with this, you can consult a dietician who uses the Glycemic Index in treating patients. See www.gifoundation.com for a list of such dieticians in your area.

Chapter 9

Start exercising

Any exercise is better than none at all. The following guidelines will help you.

◆ The best exercise for burning fat is *aerobic exercise* such as brisk walking, running, cycling, swimming, dancing, climbing stairs, cross-country running and aerobics. This kind of exercise burns lots of energy and thus body fat. (See the table on page 186.)

◆ Studies have shown that only *30 minutes of medium-intensity exercise*, such as brisk walking, three to four *times a week* will give you all the benefits discussed in the previous chapter.

◆ It's also interesting to note that *three exercise sessions of the same intensity*, each lasting 10 minutes, may be *just as effective* as a 30-minute exercise session. This makes it much easier for *all* of us to be more active in our very busy lifestyles. You could, for example, cycle for 10 minutes early morning, skip for 10 minutes before you eat your lunch, then take the dog for a 10-minute walk when you come home at night. All of us can fit short exercise sessions like these into our busy schedules.

◆ So *everybody can find the time to put in a little extra effort* to make exercise a part of any busy daily routine. Start with one 10-minute exercise session a day for the first week, and gradually increase this to three 10-minute sessions every day. Every little bit of extra activity that you make part of your life will give you all the health benefits discussed in the previous chapter.

◆ Activity levels can easily be increased by small *changes in your lifestyle*. Practise them long enough and they'll become a habit (see table below). We've given a few examples; try to add others that suit you.

Inactive lifestyle	Active lifestyle
Drive by car to the café, or from shop to shop.	Walk to the shops, or park the car in town or at a shopping centre and walk to all the shops.
Drive by car to work.	Walk or cycle to work.
Use the elevator or escalator at work, in a shopping centre or other building.	Use the stairs at work, in a shopping centre or other building.
Relax mainly in front of the TV or play computer games.	Get active; play action cricket or golf, or go dancing.
Ask others to pour you a drink.	Offer to pour drinks for everybody.
Have the gardener wash your car, keep your garden tidy, etc.	Wash your own car and do your own gardening.
Use a golf cart when playing golf.	Walk on the golf course.

Add your own personal suggestions	

◆ *Anaerobic exercise* (exercising with weights, Callanetics, Pilates, floor exercises, etc.) doesn't burn body fat to the same extent or in the same way as aerobic exercise. Anaerobic exercise improves muscle tone and, if done intensely enough, will release growth hormone, which will increase lean body mass (muscle mass), which in turn increases your basal metabolic rate, resulting in more efficient burning of body fat. Growth hormone is, however, only released when exercising at 90% maximum heart rate, i.e. at very intense exercise levels. Anaerobic exercise also decreases the risk of developing osteoporosis and heart disease. It strengthens your heart and lungs, helps to reduce stress and improves blood circulation. A combination of aerobic and anaerobic exercise offers the most benefits.

Activity and energy*			
Type of activity	Kilojoules burned in 30 minutes	Type of activity	Kilojoules burned in 30 minutes
1. Aerobic classes	466 – 1 260	10. Jogging	1 260
2. Bowls	315 – 630	11. Roller blading	735
3. Climbing stairs	630 – 1 260	12. Running	1 890
4. Cricket	504	13. Skiing (snow)	1 260
5. Cycling	1 387	14. Skipping	1 680
6. Dancing:		15. Squash	1 260
Ballet	840	16. Surfing	1 050
Modern / disco	1 260	17. Swimming	735
Ballroom dancing	840	18. Table tennis	756
National folk dancing	945	19. Tennis	924
Tap dancing	840	20. Tenpin bowling	567
7. Golf	525	21. Walking	735
8. Hockey	1 050	22. Water skiing	1 008
9. Ice skating	840	23. Windsurfing	1 050

*Table adapted from: Pollock, M L, Wilmore, J H & Fox, S M (1978): *Health and Fitness through Physical Activity*, Table 4.3 (John Wiley & Sons, Inc.); and Stoppard, M (Ed.) (1980): *The Face and Body Book*, pages 151-161 (Frances Lincoln Publishers Ltd)

Note: If you wish to follow a specialised exercise programme, it's best to consult a qualified person trained in this field. But be wary of their dietary advice; rather consult a dietician, who's the expert in nutrition. Before starting a new exercise regime, have your body fat percentage determined by a biokineticist or a dietician. Body weight may remain the same or even increase slightly as you start your exercise programme, because you'll be gaining lean body mass and losing body fat if on a slimming diet. Remember that an increase in lean body mass means an increase in your metabolic rate, as well as a slimmer body, because muscle tissue is firm and toned while fat tissue is soft and flabby. The weight gain will be temporary, unless you do heavy weight training, which results in extra muscle mass. Remember that you won't gain fat, only lean muscle mass.

Now that you've read this section, you're probably asking yourself why you didn't start exercising before. Remember that, in order to succeed, you must choose something that you enjoy, that fits into your life relatively easily, and that you can do for the rest of your life.

What are you waiting for? Start today, and enjoy it!

Recipes

Note: Recipes marked with an asterisk (*) were taken from *Eating for Sustained Energy*, by Liesbet Delport and Gabi Steenkamp (Tafelberg, 2000)

Nutritional analysis of the recipes

The Box: You will notice that there is a box containing nutritional information ith every recipe.

All values have been rounded off to the nearest whole number.

It contains the following information and reflects the **amounts per serving**:

Glycemic Index (GI) – this is a calculated value. The value in real life will probably be lower, due to the interaction of the different nutrients with one another. The GI gives an indication of how fast and by how much the portion of food will affect blood glucose levels.

Fat (g) – This value reflects the total fat content of the serving per person. Although the saturated fat and cholesterol content is not displayed, these are also kept low.

Carbohydrates (g) – This value gives the total carbohydrate content per serving and includes the carbohydrate present in the dairy, starch, vegetables and fruit.

Fibre (g) – This is the total amount of fibre per serving, including both soluble and insoluble fibre.

Protein (g) - This represents the total amount of protein per serving.

Kilojoules (kJ) – This is the total kilojoule value (energy) per serving (to obtain calories, simply divide by 4,2).

After the box, in each recipe, the contents per serving are given.

For example: One serving is equivalent to **1 Starch** and **1 Protein**.

The **nutritional contents of 1 portion for each food group** are as follows:

Dairy - the analysis for a low-fat Dairy portion applies.

530 kJ, 8 g protein, 5 g fat and 12 g carbohydrate.

When applicable, the analysis of a fatfree Dairy portion was used.

340 kJ, 8 g protein, 0 g fat and 12 g carbohydrate.

Protein – the analysis for a low-fat Protein portion applies.

328 kJ, 7 g protein and 5,5 g fat.

Starch – a Starch portion implies the following:

289 kJ, 15 g carbohydrate, 2 g protein and traces of fat.

Fat – a Fat portion implies the following:

190 kJ and 5 g fat.

Vegetables – The kilojoules, carbohydrates and protein contained in a limited Vegetable portion are:

119 kJ, 7 g carbohydrates and 2 g protein.

When the other food group portions in a recipe accounted for the total allowable kilojoule content, we did not count the kilojoules of the limited vegetables, even if the recipe contained some limited vegetable. Free vegetables contain less than 105 kJ per 100 g vegetables.

Fruit – a Fruit portion implies the following:

170 kJ and 10 g carbohydrate.

Apple crumble*
Serves 6

1 x 410 g tin pie apples
10 ml lemon juice (2 t)
30 ml raw honey (2 T)
50 ml flour (3 T + 1 t)
250 ml oat bran (1 C)
50 ml lite margarine (3 T + 1 t)
50 ml soft brown sugar (3 T + 1 t)
1 ml salt ($^1/_4$ t)

Nutrients per serving
Glycemic Index 56
(Intermediate GI)
Fat 5 g
Carbohydrate 30 g
Protein 2 g
kJ 771
Fibre 3 g

1. Place the pie apples in a greased pie dish, and pour the lemon juice and honey over.
2. Rub together flour, oat bran, margarine, brown sugar and salt and sprinkle this mixture over the apples.
3. Bake in the oven at 180 °C, until crust is brown.
4. Serve with fat-reduced cream or custard made with low-fat milk (page 198), if desired.

Dietician's notes:
◆ This is a moist and flavourful apple crumble that's equally delicious without any low-fat custard.
◆ The nutritional analysis is for the crumble only, without the low-fat custard.
◆ A good dessert for carbo-loading, high in carbohydrates and low enough in protein and fat.
◆ Remember that raw honey has a lower GI than commercial honey.

One serving is equivalent to: $1^1/_2$ starch + 1 fruit +1 fat

Brinjal pâté

Makes 500 ml (2 C)

Serves 10

500 g brinjals (1 large or 3 medium-
  sized brinjals;
also called aubergines or eggplant)
15 – 20 ml lemon juice (3 – 4 t)
4 cloves garlic, crushed
4 dried apricots, soaked in a little
  warm water
15 ml peanut butter (1 T)
2 ml sesame oil ($^1/_2$ t)
salt to taste
chilli powder to taste
60 ml fat-free yoghurt (4 T)
15 ml chopped parsley (1 T)
30 ml fresh coriander, chopped (2 T)
5 ml ground cumin (1 t)

Nutrients per 50 ml serving
(50 ml = 3 T)
Glycemic Index <40
(Low GI)
Fat 1 g
Carbohydrate 3 g
Protein 1 g
kJ 115
Fibre 1 g

1. Wash and prick the whole brinjals; do not peel.
2. Bake in the oven at 180 °C until tender, 45 – 50 minutes, *or* microwave on high for 11 minutes, until soft.
3. Allow to cool, then peel.
4. Place the brinjal flesh, lemon juice, garlic, softened apricots, peanut butter and sesame oil in a food processor and purée until smooth.
5. Remove from the food processor, season to taste with salt and chilli powder and stir in the yoghurt, parsley, coriander and cumin.
6. Serve as a snack or starter with low-GI biscuits such as Provita.

Dietician's notes:
◆ This pâté also makes a lovely dip. Serve with vegetable crudités and low-fat pretzels.
◆ This makes a perfect low-GI, low-fat spread for low-GI crackers and sandwiches.
◆ Used in such small quantities, it contains negligible kilojoules.

One serving (50 ml) is equivalent to: 1 limited vegetable

Bran muffins*

Makes 24 large muffins
Note: This batter has to stand overnight.

Nutrients per muffin
Glycemic Index 58
(Intermediate GI)
Fat 3 g
Carbohydrate 22 g
Protein 3 g
Fibre 3 g
kJ 507

2 eggs
150 g soft brown sugar (1 C)
60 ml canola oil (4 T)
250 ml oat bran, pressed down into the cup (1 C)
375 ml flour, sifted before measuring (1½ C)
500 ml digestive bran (2 C)
2 ml salt (½ t)
15 ml bicarbonate of soda (1 T)
5 ml ground cinnamon (1 t)
1 large apple, grated
250 ml sultanas (1 C)
500 ml low-fat or skimmed milk (2 C)
5 ml vanilla essence (1 t)

1. Beat together eggs, sugar and oil.
2. Add all the dry ingredients, grated apple and the sultanas.
3. Mix the milk and vanilla and add to the flour mixture.
4. Stir until well blended, but do not overmix as this raises the GI.
5. Leave overnight in the fridge.
6. When ready to bake, stir and drop into muffin pans.
7. Bake at 180 °C for 15 minutes.

◆ This mixture can be kept in the fridge for up to 30 days. Do not freeze the batter.
◆ Baked muffins freeze very well.

Dietician's notes:
◆ These muffins are deliciously moist and don't need margarine or butter.
◆ Despite all the oat bran and bran (we've loaded the muffins as much as we could, without sacrificing texture), the GI is still 58. It's the *flour* that does this, *not* the sugar. Even if we halve the sugar, the GI doesn't come down. Interesting!
◆ If low-fat yoghurt, plain or fruit, is used instead of milk, the GI is lowered to 55.

One muffin is equivalent to: 1 starch + ½ fat + 1 fruit

Carrot cake*
Serves 12

180 g lite margarine (200 ml)
250 ml castor sugar (1 C)
250 ml cake flour (1 C), sifted before
    measuring
pinch of salt
7 ml ground cinnamon ($1\frac{1}{2}$ t)
2 ml ground nutmeg ($\frac{1}{2}$ t)
pinch of ground cloves
10 ml baking powder (2 t)
5 ml bicarbonate of soda (1 t)
250 ml oat bran (1 C)
3 eggs, using 2 whole eggs and 1 egg white
125 ml grated carrot ($\frac{1}{2}$ C; 1 large or 2 small)
1 apple, grated
150 ml sultanas ($\frac{3}{5}$ C)

ICING
250 g low-fat or fat-free cottage cheese
60 ml icing sugar (4 T)
5 ml vanilla essence (1 t)

Nutrients per slice with icing
Glycemic Index 61 (Intermediate GI)
Fat 10 g
Carbohydrate 37 g
Protein 7 g
kJ 1 102
Fibre 2 g

1. Cream margarine and sugar for no more than 3 minutes.
2. Sift flour, salt, spices, baking powder and bicarbonate of soda in a separate bowl. Add the oat bran, lifting up the mixture with a spoon to incorporate air.
3. Add eggs and egg white, one by one, to the margarine and sugar, adding 30 – 45 ml (2 – 3 T) of the flour mixture with each egg. Beat for no more than 1 minute after adding each egg.
4. Add the rest of the flour mixture and stir dry ingredients into the egg mixture by hand, using a wooden spoon.
5. Fold in raw carrots, apple and sultanas.
6. Place in a greased 25 cm round cake tin and bake at 160 °C for 30 – 45 minutes.
7. When cool, ice with cottage cheese icing.
8. Icing: Mix the cottage cheese with the icing sugar and vanilla essence taking care not to overmix. Spread over the top of the cake.

Dietician's notes:
- It's very important not to overmix this cake, as this would make it more easily digestible and thereby raise the GI.
- The cottage cheese icing helps to lower the GI value.
- Without the icing, the GI would be 62 and the energy would drop slightly to 1 039 kJ per portion.

One serving, with icing, is equivalent to: 2 starch + 2 fat + 1 fruit

Crumpets*

Makes about 20 crumpets (6 cm in diameter)

Nutrients per crumpet
Glycemic Index 60 (Intermediate GI)
Fat 1 g
Carbohydrate 8 g
Protein 2 g
kJ 213
Fibre 0,6 g

1 egg, lightly beaten
10 ml sugar (2 t)
2 ml salt ($^1/_2$ t)
250 ml low-fat or fat-free milk (1 C)
5 ml canola or sunflower oil (1 t)
250 ml cake flour, sifted before measuring (1 C)
5 ml bicarbonate of soda (1 t)
5 ml baking powder (1 t)
125 ml oat bran ($^1/_2$ C)
1 large apple, grated with the skin

1. Beat the egg in a mixing bowl, using a hand whisk.
2. Add the sugar and salt and beat for no more than 1 minute.
3. Add half the milk and the oil. Beat for no more than 1 minute.
4. Sift together the flour, bicarbonate and baking powder and stir gradually into the egg and milk mixture, with a wooden spoon, until smooth and lump-free. Do not overmix.
5. Add the rest of the milk, the oat bran and the grated apple and mix gently.
6. Leave the batter to stand for 10 minutes to moisten all the ingredients.
7. Heat a non-stick frying pan and spray with cooking spray.
8. Ladle about 4 separate tablespoons (4 x 15 ml) batter into pan and cook the 4 crumpets over moderately high heat until bubbly on top and light brown underneath.
9. Turn crumpets to brown other side.
10. Repeat with the remaining batter.

Dietician's notes:

◆ There's no need to spread margarine or butter on these crumpets. Eat dry with a little marmalade or apricot jam and lower-fat cheese, if desired.

◆ Be careful not to beat the batter too much. Beating improves digestibility, which would *increase the GI* of the crumpets.

◆ It's *very important to add the apple*, as this is the vital ingredient that lowers the GI of the crumpets.

One crumpet is equivalent to: $^1/_2$ starch

Custard, low fat*

Makes 4 x 125 ml servings ($^1/_2$ C) or
  8 x 62,5 ml servings ($^1/_4$ C)

500 ml low-fat or skimmed milk (2 C)
30 ml sugar (2 T)
30 ml custard powder (2 T)
5 ml vanilla essence (1 t)

Nutrients per serving (125 ml)
Glycemic Index 52 (Low GI)
Fat 2 g
Carbohydrate 15 g
Protein 4 g
kJ 416
Fibre negligible

1. Bring 400 ml ($1^3/_5$ C) of the milk to boil.
2. While the milk is heating up, place the reserved 100 ml ($^2/_5$ C) of the milk, plus the sugar, in a small bowl and mix to dissolve the sugar. Add the custard powder and stir to a smooth paste.
3. Just as the milk begins to bubble, pour half of it into the custard powder mixture, and stir.
4. Pour this back into the saucepan of hot milk and bring to the boil, stirring.
5. Cook until thickened.
6. Add vanilla essence, if desired.
7. Serve cold with low-GI pudding.

To make banana custard, use half a banana per person with 125 ml ($^1/_2$ C) cold custard. The GI then rises by one point, to 53. Remember to omit one of your fruit snacks.

Dietician's notes:
- In the GI tables used in Australia, the GI of custard is given as 43. We haven't yet tested the GI of custard in South Africa, so the value given here is the *calculated value*, based on the recipe ingredients.
- We feel quite sure that the true tested GI of custard will be lower than the calculated value, due to the interaction of the nutrients with each other, especially when eaten cold.
- It's important to eat the custard *cold*.
- When custard is hot, it has a higher GI value than when it's cold, as a result of a change in the crystal structure of the cooked starch when it cools down. The starch, in this case, is the custard powder.

Diabetics please note that this low-fat custard, if eaten cold, is quite safe and will not suddenly raise your blood glucose levels. This custard is low GI, despite the sugar it contains.

One 125 ml ($^1/_2$ C) serving is equivalent to: 1 starch + $^1/_2$ dairy
One 62,5 ml ($^1/_4$ C) serving is equivalent to: 1 starch

Date and oat muffins*
Makes 12 muffins

250 ml wholewheat flour (1 C)
250 ml oat bran (1 C)
10 ml baking powder (2 t)
2 ml ground cinnamon ($^1/_2$ t)
1 ml ground nutmeg ($^1/_4$ t)
1 ml ground cloves ($^1/_4$ t)
45 ml lite margarine (3 T)
1 large apple, peeled and grated
125 ml dates, chopped ($^1/_2$ C)
150 ml skimmed milk ($^3/_5$ C)
15 ml brown sugar (1T)
2 egg whites, whisked to soft-peak stage

Nutrients per muffin
Glycemic Index 60
(Intermediate GI)
Fat 3 g
Carbohydrate 20 g
Protein 4 g
kJ 533
Fibre 3 g

1. Preheat the oven to 200 °C.
2. Sift the flour and add back the bran.
3. Add the oat bran, baking powder, cinnamon, nutmeg and cloves.
4. Gently mix with a spoon, lifting up the flour mixture to incorporate air.
5. Rub in the margarine.
6. Add apples and dates and mix well.
7. Add milk and brown sugar and stir.
8. Fold in the egg whites.
9. Spoon into sprayed muffin pans.
10. Bake in preheated oven for 15 – 20 minutes.

Dietician's note:
◆ Compare this recipe with the bran muffins (page 193), where we use a whole cup of sugar. They have a lower GI value! We hope this convinces you that sugar isn't always the baddie we all thought it was.

One muffin is equivalent to: 1 starch + $^1/_2$ fat + 1 fruit

Fat-free salad dressing

Makes 200 ml (4/5 C)
Serves 10

60 ml raw honey (4 T)
60 ml balsamic vinegar (4 T)
60 ml whole-grain mustard (4 T)

Nutrients per serving (20 ml)
Glycemic Index 55 (Low GI)
Fat negligible
Carbohydrate 7 g
Protein negligible
kJ 137

1. Heat the honey in a glass jar until runny (about 30 seconds on high in a micro-wave).
2. Add the vinegar and mustard.
3. Shake in the jar until very thick.
4. Spoon 20 ml (4 t) per person onto salad.

Dietician's notes:

◆ The calculated GI of this dressing seems quite high because of the honey. However, the vinegar will bring the GI down in real life, so this is a wonderful, fat-free, low-GI dressing.

◆ Remember it's important to use *raw* honey, as other honey has a high GI.

One serving (20 ml) is equivalent to: $^1/_2$ starch

(Adapted from Tabitha Hume's recipe)

Fish burger patties*
Makes 6 patties

1 x 410 g tin salmon, or pilchards in
    tomato sauce
1 medium onion, finely grated
10 ml finely chopped parsley (2 t)
250 ml low-GI oats, e.g. Bokomo,
    Woolworths, Pick 'n Pay (1 C)
1 egg
5 ml canola or olive oil (1 t)

Nutrients per fish patty
Glycemic Index <30
(Low GI)
Fat 6 g
Carbohydrate 3 g
Protein 14 g
kJ 511
Fibre negligible

1. Remove fish from the sauce and flake.
2. Add the onion, parsley, oats, egg and some of the sauce to make a firm batter. Be careful not to overmix.
3. Shape the mixture into 6 large fish cakes or patties.
4. Heat the oil and fry the patties quickly on both sides.
5. Serve on a hamburger roll spread with low-fat (lite) mayonnaise.
6. Add some shredded lettuce, bean sprouts, tomato sauce and top with a slice of pineapple for extra zing.

◆ A quick and easy dish that's easy on the pocket as well.
◆ Because the GI of the patties is so low, the fish burger can be enjoyed with an ordinary bread roll.
◆ Remember not to butter the roll, to keep the fat content down. Use only a little lite mayonnaise, tomato sauce, mustard and/or chutney.
◆ Serve with a low-GI salad.

Dietician's note:
Pilchards are a rich source of Omega-3 essential fatty acids. Modern diets are usually lacking in Omega-3 fatty acids, so this is a pleasant way to include such a rich source once a week. Omega-3 fatty acids are especially important for allergy-prone people and those with compromised immune systems. They've also been shown to be beneficial for ADHD and heart disease.

One fish patty is equivalent to: 2 protein

Fruit salad*

Serves 6

1 small papino
1 small green apple
1 small red apple
3 oranges
1 banana
1 kiwifruit
10 large grapes
10 ml sugar (optional) (2 t)
30 ml freshly squeezed lemon juice (2 T)

Nutrients per serving
Glycemic index 47
(Without sugar)
(Low GI)
Fat 0
Carbohydrate 23 g
Protein 1 g
kJ 439
Fibre 4 g

1. Peel papino, remove the pips and cut flesh into cubes.
2. Quarter the apples (don't peel), remove the core and then chop the flesh into cubes.
3. Peel the oranges as you would an apple and then, using a sharp knife, slide the blade of the knife between the segments and push the flesh out into a bowl. You should end up with whole peeled segments.
4. Peel and slice the banana.
5. Peel the kiwifruit, cut in half lengthways, then slice thickly.
6. Cut each grape in half and remove the pips.
7. Mix all the fruit together, add the lemon juice and the sugar if desired and mix thoroughly.
8. Chill before serving.

Dietician's notes:

◆ Adding lemon juice lowers the GI of the fruit salad even further.
◆ With the sugar, the GI of the whole fruit salad is 48. The reason for this is that the fruit has a lower GI than the sugar, so the sugar with the higher GI would slightly increase the total GI. But even at 48, the GI is quite acceptable, even for diabetics.

One serving is equivalent to: 2 fruit

(See page 204 for the Glycemic Index of fruits)

The Glycemic Index of fruits
Tropical fruits have intermediate GI values. (See GI tables at back of book.)
Deciduous and citrus fruits have low GI values. (See GI tables at back of book.)
The more *tart (sour)* a fruit, the lower its GI.
Melons are the only high GI fruits, and should therefore not be eaten on their own.

Grilled seed loaf Cheezie

Serves 1

1 slice seed loaf or wheat-free rye bread
15 ml hummus* (1 T)
10 ml grated cheddar cheese (2 t)
2 ml grated Parmesan cheese ($\frac{1}{2}$ t)

Nutrients per cheezie
Glycemic Index 49
(Low GI)
Fat 3 g
Carbohydrate 21 g
Protein 7 g
kJ 576
Fibre 3 g

1. Spread hummus thickly on sliced seed loaf.
2. Sprinkle cheeses on top.
3. Grill until bubbly.

* Bought or homemade – see recipe on page 207.

Dietician's note:
◆ Seed loaf is not suitable for those suffering from irritable bowel syndrome (spastic colon). Use wheat-free rye bread instead.
◆ Cheddar and Parmesan are high-fat cheeses. If you want to use more cheese, rather use lower-fat cheese such as mozzarella.

One cheezie is equivalent to: 1 starch + 1 protein/dairy

Healthy breakfast muffins

Makes 15 large muffins that are a meal on their own

125 ml sultanas ($^1/_2$ C)
125 ml oat bran ($^1/_2$ C)
125 ml wholewheat flour/ Nutty Wheat ($^1/_2$ C)
125 ml wholewheat Pronutro ($^1/_2$ C)
125 ml low-GI oats, e.g. Bokomo, Woolworths, Pick 'n Pay ($^1/_2$ C)
125 ml Hi Fibre Bran ($^1/_2$ C)
125 ml cake flour ($^1/_2$ C)
250 ml digestive bran (1 C)
2 ml salt ($^1/_2$ t)
5 ml baking powder (1 t)
7,5 ml bicarbonate of soda ($1^1/_2$ t)
1 small Granny Smith apple or firm pear, grated (100 g)
1 small raw sweet potato, grated (125 g)
1 egg, separated
5 ml vanilla essence (1 t)
30 ml canola oil (2 T)
125 ml soft brown sugar ($^1/_2$ C)
375 ml fat-free milk ($1^1/_2$ C)
1 egg white

Nutrients per muffin
Glycemic Index 57
(Intermediate GI)
Fat 3 g
Carbohydrate 23 g
Protein 4 g
kJ 599
Fibre 5 g

1. Heat oven to 220 °C.
2. Mix all the dry ingredients, add the grated apple and grated sweet potato.
3. Mix gently and set aside.
4. Beat the egg yolk, vanilla essence, oil and sugar in a large bowl.
5. Add the dry ingredients, alternating with the milk.
6. Mix gently, but thoroughly.
7. Beat the egg whites until stiff and fold into batter.
8. Spoon into muffin pans and put into oven.
9. Turn oven down to 180 °C and bake for 20 – 25 minutes.
10. Insert a skewer in centre of 1 muffin to check whether the muffins are done.
11. If there's raw batter on the skewer, bake for another 5 minutes.

Dietician's notes:

◆ These muffins are particularly high in soluble fibre, which is good for a healthy bowel, lowering cholesterol, blood glucose levels, and insulin response.

◆ Eat the muffins on the same day, as they don't keep well because of their high moisture content, or freeze and defrost individually as needed.

◆ White cake flour can be substituted for the wholewheat flour if you prefer a less bran-filled muffin.

◆ The GI of wholewheat flour and cake flour is the same.

One muffin is equivalent to: $1^1/_2$ starch + $^1/_2$ fat

Some interesting facts about sweet potatoes

Sweet potatoes are root vegetables that are often confused with the yam, but they're tastier and more nutritious. They lower the GI of any dish, especially when used instead of potatoes. African herbalists have used sweet potatoes for their powerful medicinal properties for generations and the vegetable is thought to be useful in the treatment of cancer. Sweet potatoes are also great oven roasted, microwaved and in flan, quiche or pie recipes (see recipe on page 210).

Hummus

Makes 500 ml (2 C)

Serves 8

1 x 410g can chickpeas

60 ml lemon juice

1 – 2 cloves fresh garlic, crushed (5 – 10 ml [1 – 2 t])

60 ml tahini (sesame seed paste) (4 T)

salt

pepper

paprika

parsley

Nutrients per serving (60 ml)

Glycemic Index <30 (Low GI)

Fat 4 g

Carbohydrate 8 g

Protein 4 g

kJ 349

Fibre 2 g

1. Mix all the ingredients in a liquidiser or food processor and season to taste.
2. Store in the fridge for up to one week.

Dietician's notes

◆ This makes a lovely lower-fat spread for sandwiches, in place of margarine or butter.

◆ Hummus is also delicious as a dip for vegetable crudités and pretzels, or as a side dish at a picnic.

One serving is equivalent to: $^1/_2$ starch + $^1/_2$ protein

Mushroom sauce

Serves 4 as a sauce for meat
Serves 2 as a pasta sauce

250 g mushrooms (1 punnet)
'₂ medium onion
1 clove garlic
5 ml canola or olive oil (1 t)
125 ml skimmed milk ($^1/_2$ C)
5 ml flour (1 t)
5 ml oat bran (1 t)
45 ml water (3 T)
2 ml salt ($^1/_2$ t)
freshly ground black pepper

**Nutrients per serving
(as a meat sauce)**
Glycemic index <30
(Low GI)
Fat 2 g
Carbohydrate 6 g
Protein 3 g
kJ 202
Fibre 1 g

1. Wipe mushrooms clean with a paper towel or wash them, if they're dirty.
2. Finely chop the onion and garlic.
3. Heat the oil in a frying pan. When hot, add the onion and garlic.
4. Gently fry over medium heat until onions are transparent, then add the mushrooms.
5. Pour milk over, turn heat down and simmer for 10 minutes.
6. Mix flour and oat bran, then moisten with water to make a smooth, runny paste.
7. Pour flour mixture into milk and mushrooms, stirring all the time. Bring to boil and cook until sauce has thickened.
8. Season with salt and pepper.

Dietician's notes

◆ Remember, whenever you thicken a sauce, oat bran can be used in combination with the high-GI flour to lower the GI, as we have done in this recipe.

◆ This sauce can also be used as a pasta sauce. The recipe then serves 2.

◆ For variation, you can also add 100 g lean, chopped ham or cooked chicken. Count two extra meat portions per person.

◆ Serve with pasta and a large salad, and you have a perfectly balanced meal.

One portion pasta sauce (serves 2) is equivalent to: 1 starch + 1 limited vegetable

One portion sauce for meat (serves 4) is equivalent to: 1 limited vegetable

Roast sweet potatoes and butternut
Serves 4

2 medium-sized sweet potatoes (at least 200 g each)

$^1/_2$ small butternut, peeled and diced (not more than 200 g)

canola or olive oil

5 ml rosemary, dried or fresh (1 t)

Nutrients per serving
Glycemic Index 56 (Intermediate GI)
Fat 2 g
Carbohydrate 27 g
Protein 2 g
kJ 616
Fibre 5 g

1. Preheat the oven to 200 °C.
2. Cook the sweet potatoes in their jackets in a microwave oven, or boil in water on the stove, until just done, but still firm.
3. Peel and slice the butternut into thick rings.
4. Microwave or cook the butternut until just done.
5. Peel the sweet potatoes and cut into large chunks.
6. Pour about 25 ml oil (5 t) into a flat baking pan and place in the hot oven.
7. As soon as the oil is hot (about 5 minutes) remove the baking pan from the oven and pour out *all* the oil.
8. Place the cooked sweet potatoes and butternut in the baking pan and turn the vegetables until they're completely covered in a thin layer of oil.
9. Sprinkle with the rosemary.
10. Roast, turning once, until evenly browned.
11. Serve with a mixed salad (no carrots or beetroot) and a small portion of lean, grilled meat, fish or chicken.

Dietician's notes
◆ Potatoes have a high GI, but sweet potatoes have a low GI. For this reason, we've included a low-fat method of roasting sweet potatoes.
◆ Butternut hasn't been tested for its GI, but because the only internationally tested GI value we have for yellow pumpkin is high, the quantity of butternut you use should be half that of the sweet potato (note quantities in recipe).
◆ Both sweet potatoes and butternut have a good fibre content.

One portion is equivalent to: $1^1/_2$ starch + 1 limited vegetable

Three-bean salad*

Serves 12

Nutrients per serving
Glycemic Index 44
(Low GI)
Fat 1 g
Carbohydrate 11 g
Protein 4 g
kJ 322
Fibre 5 g

1 x 410 g tin butter beans, drained
1 x 410 g tin baked beans in tomato sauce
1 x 410 g tin French-cut green beans,
   drained
15 ml sugar (1 T)
2 ml mustard powder ($^1/_2$ t)
15 ml canola or olive oil (1 T)
100 ml white or brown vinegar ($^2/_5$ C)
15 ml fresh basil (1 T) or 5 ml dried (1 t)
freshly ground black pepper to taste

1. Mix the three tins of beans.
2. Place the sugar, mustard powder, oil, vinegar and basil in a sauce-pan and heat until the sugar has dissolved. Stir continuously.
3. Pour the sauce over the bean mixture.
4. Season with pepper to taste and mix well.
5. Chill for at least three hours, but preferably overnight.
6. Serve cold.

Dietician's notes
◆ This is a low-fat, high-fibre salad that goes well with all outdoor meals.
◆ Three-bean salad keeps for up to two weeks, in a sealed container, in the fridge.
◆ It's ideal for making in advance for picnics, or for camping and self-catering holidays.

Half a portion is equal to: 1 limited vegetable
One portion is equivalent to: $^1/_2$ starch + 1 limited vegetable

Tomato sauce for pasta

Serves 4

Nutrients per serving (sauce only)
Glycemic Index <30 (Low GI)
Fat 3 g
Carbohydrate 19 g
Protein 7 g
kJ 628
Fibre 7 g

5 ml canola or olive oil (1 t)
2 rashers lean bacon, fat removed, and chopped
2 medium-sized onions, chopped
5 ml crushed garlic (1 t) or 2 cloves garlic
1 carrot, peeled and coarsely grated
1 green pepper, seeded and chopped
4 ripe tomatoes, peeled and diced
5 ml thyme (1 t)
5 ml origanum (1 t)
30 ml fresh basil (2 T) or 5 ml dried (1 t)
2 ml salt ($^1/_2$ t)
freshly ground black pepper to taste
70 g canned tomato paste
$^1/_2$ x 410 g tin butter beans, drained and coarsely mashed
20 ml grated Parmesan cheese (4 t)

1. Heat the oil in a large saucepan and gently fry the bacon, onions, garlic, carrot and green pepper until the onions are transparent. If they start to burn, add 15 – 30 ml (1 – 2 T) water and stir.
2. Add the diced tomatoes and simmer for 5 minutes.
3. Add the herbs, salt, pepper, tomato paste and mashed beans and simmer for a further 5 minutes.
4. Spoon over freshly cooked pasta of your choice on a serving dish and sprinkle with Parmesan cheese.
5. Serve immediately with either two cooked vegetables or a tossed salad.

Dietician's notes
◆ Note the high fibre content, because of the beans in the sauce.
◆ This meal is ideal for carbo-loading as it contains long-acting carbohydrates and not too much fat and protein.
◆ The GI of carrots is generally high, but in this recipe combining it with the beans and other low-GI vegetables cancels out its effect.

One serving (sauce only) is equivalent to: 1 protein/dairy + 1 limited vegetable + free vegetables

Vegetable sauce for pasta

Serves 4

Nutrients per serving
Glycemic Index <40
(Low GI)
Fat 3 g
Carbohydrate 29 g
Protein 9 g
kJ 739
Fibre 11 g

5 ml canola or olive oil (1 t)
2 small onions, chopped
10 ml minced garlic (2 t)
250 g sliced mushrooms (1 punnet)
$^1/_2$ green pepper, seeded and chopped
1 carrot, grated
100 g broccoli, cut into small florets (1 C)
1 x 410 g tin baked beans in tomato sauce, lightly mashed
15 ml tomato purée (1 T)
5 ml mixed herbs (1 t)
125 ml low-fat milk ($^1/_2$ C)
pinch of ground nutmeg
2 ml salt ($^1/_2$ t)
freshly ground black pepper to taste

1. Heat the oil in a non-stick frying pan.
2. Add the onions and garlic and cook for about 5 minutes.
3. Add the mushrooms, green pepper and carrot. Cook for a further 5 minutes.
4. Add the broccoli, baked beans, tomato purée and herbs.
5. Stir in the milk and nutmeg.
6. Simmer for 15 minutes.
7. Once sauce has thickened slightly, season with salt and pepper.
8. Serve on freshly cooked pasta of your choice.

Dietician's notes

◆ This dish has an exceptionally high fibre content and is also very low in fat.
◆ Since the beans are mashed in this sauce, it is also ideal for those suffering from irritable bowel syndrome.
◆ The nutritional analysis is for the sauce only. Remember that 125 ml ($^1/_2$ C) cooked pasta (30 g raw) is equivalent to 1 starch.

One serving is equivalent to: 1 protein + 1 limited vegetable + free vegetables

Vegetable soup
Serves 4

5 ml Carotino, olive or canola oil (1 t)
1 medium-sized onion, finely chopped
2 cloves garlic, chopped
1 large carrot, grated
1 leek, washed and sliced
250 ml broccoli, chopped (1 C)
1 vegetable stock cube, dissolved in
    1 litre (4 C) boiling water
1 x 410 g tin baked beans in tomato sauce

Nutrients per serving (about 2 ladles of soup)
Glycemic Index <40 (Low GI)
Fat 2 g
Carbohydrate 28 g
Protein 8g
kJ 710
Fibre 12 g

1. Heat oil in a large saucepan.
2. Add onion, garlic, carrot and leek and stir-fry for 10 minutes.
3. Add broccoli and stir.
4. Add stock cube dissolved in hot water.
5. Add baked beans and bring to boil.
6. Simmer for 5 minutes.
7. Serve with Grilled seed loaf cheezie (recipe on page 204) or Apple crumble (recipe on page 191).

Dietician's notes
◆ Remember to choose between the cheezie and the apple crumble.
◆ This soup has a very high fibre content as well as a lovely low GI. All the vitamins and minerals from the vegetables make this a really healthy meal.

One serving is equivalent to: 1 protein + 1 limited vegetable + free vegetables

Carotino oil
Palm oil, marketed in South Africa as Carotino oil, is bright orange in colour, and is particularly high in vitamin E and beta-carotene. The beta-carotene is what gives the oil its bright orange colour. Palm oil is not the same as palm kernel oil. Palm kernel oil, a saturated fat, should be limited in our diet. Palm oil, on the other hand, contains 50% mono-unsaturated fats, and is thus a healthy oil. But, since it is still 100% fat, only small quantities should be used, as in this recipe.

GI logos and lists

Note: Comprehensive GI lists giving actual values are available in book form from GIFSA at www.gifoundation.com

Endorsement logo's of the Glycemic Index Foundation of South Africa (GIFSA)

Low Fat, Low GI

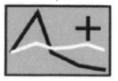

Frequent Foods

The **Green Plus** GIFSA logo means that the product or food endorsed with this logo is low in fat ($\leq$ 3g fat/100g food), has a low GI value ($\leq$ 40) and can be consumed frequently.

Lower Fat, Low GI

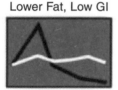

Often Foods

The **Green** GIFSA logo means that the product or food endorsed with this logo is lower in fat (3,1 g-10 g fat/food), has a low GI value ($\leq$ 55) and can be consumed often.

Lower Fat, Intermediate GI

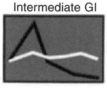

Special Treats

The **Orange** GIFSA logo means that the product of food endorsed with this logo is lower in fat than its regular counterpart, has an intermediate GI value ($\leq$ 69) and can be eaten as a special treat. The fat is always controlled to a maximum of 15g/100g.

Lower Fat, High GI

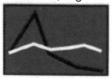

Best after exercise

The **Red** GIFSA logo means that the product or food endorsed with this logo is lower in fat than its regular counterpart, has a high GI value ($\geq$70) and is best eaten after exercise lasting at least one hour (two hours for diabetics). The fat is always controlled to a maximum of 15g/100g.

Glycemic Index list according to food groups

Items are listed according to food groups, in order and from lowest to highest GI, using glucose as the reference food.

Key

bold	These products have been tested in South Africa by GIFSA
*	High fat foods. These products do not comply with GIFSA's and the Heart Foundation of South Africa's standard's for a lower-fat product.
Calculated	Theoretical calculation done by Liesbet Delport (ED) and Gabi Steenkamp (GS)
Estimated	Estimated values based on extensive experience in GI testing and developing low-GI, lower-fat recipes (by ED and GS).

Low GI (55 and below)

Dairy

All low-fat and fat-free milk (plain and sweetened)

Full-cream milk*

Low-fat buttermilk (check labels!)

Buttermilk, full-cream*

All low-fat and fat-free yoghurt (plain and sweetened)

Fat-free Muesli Corner and Strawberry Corner, sweetened with fructose (Clover Danone)

Cooled low-fat and fat-free custard (sweetened with sugar)

Hot low-fat and fat-free custard (unsweetened/artificially sweetened)

Fine Form Chocolate Ice cream

Low-fat and fat-free ice cream, milk-based (sweetened and unsweetened), e.g. **Dialite**

Cereals

Wholewheat Pronutro, Original and Apple Bake (Bokomo) with or without low-fat/fat-free milk

Hi-Fibre Bran (Kelloggs)

Shredded Bran (Pick 'n Pay No Name Brand)

Sorghum with added acid, i.e. lemon juice or vinegar (South African)

Nature's Source range of low-GI muesli, i.e. Mixed Berries, Orange & Spices, and Apple and Cinnamon

Maximize cereal (Bokomo)

Cooled mealiemeal porridge

Oat bran, raw (Jungle)

All-bran Flakes (Kelloggs) with skimmed milk

Fine Form Muesli

Morning Harvest Muesli (Bokomo)

Pronutro Original, with low-fat milk

Raw muesli containing mainly oats (preferably Bokomo/Woolworths/ Pick 'n Pay No Name Brand), oat bran, digestive bran, wheatgerm, Hi-fibre Bran/Shredded Bran, Wholewheat Pronutro, sultanas and a few nuts (not Brazil nuts!)

Bread and flour

Bran Crisp Bread

Provita wholewheat crackers (Original and Multigrain)

Fine Form sliced brown bread; whole-grain rye bread (pumpernickel); **Uncle Salie's Homemade Brown Seed Loaf** (Sasko); and any other bread containing lots of whole barley, rye, wheat, buckwheat, crushed wheat, oats (preferably Bokomo/Woolworths/Pick 'n Pay No Name Brand), oat bran, digestive bran, soya/pea flour, low-fat dairy and/or low GI fruit, e.g. sultanas

Fruit bread, e.g. raisin bread, banana bread

Soya and pea flour

Oat bran (Jungle), raw. Digestive bran, rice bran

Starches

All legumes, i.e. dried and cooked or canned beans, peas, lentils, pea dhal, etc., including soya beans, baked beans, chickpeas, etc. (sweetened and unsweetened); low-fat soups made with legumes; stew made from dried beans

Pearled (whole) barley and cracked barley

Whole and cracked rye

Cooled samp

Pearled wholewheat/Weet-rice/Bulgur wheat/Stampkoring, crushed wheat and buckwheat

All pasta (macaroni, spaghetti and noodles; plain, wholewheat and spinach) made from 100% durum wheat or durum wheat semolina, e.g. **Fine Form pasta, Mr Pasta & Pasta Grande Spaghetti** and low-fat instant pasta (durum wheat; *not* 2-Minute Noodles)

Cooled mealiemeal

Tastic rice

Sweet potato (Australian)

Long-grain rice (Canadian)

Wild rice (Canadian)

Whole corn (canned and frozen) and corn on the cob/sweetcorn (fresh)

Brown rice with lentils (calculated using equal quantities of rice and lentils)

Fruit

All fresh and dried deciduous fruit, i.e. apricots, fresh cherries, peaches, nectarines, plums, pears and apples, as well as strawberries. Note that stone fruits and temperate climate fruits have lower GI values. Note: Watch portion sizes of dried fruits, as they are very concentrated.

All citrus fruit, i.e. oranges, naartjies, grapefruit, limes, lemons and unsweetened citrus peel. Note: The more tart/sharp/acid the fruit, the lower the GI value.

Kiwifruit and grapes (watch portion sizes!)

Canned apples – estimated

Canned pears (in fruit juice)

Canned peaches (in fruit juice)

Canned apricots (in fruit juice) – estimated

Canned fruit salad (Canadian)

Fruit juices: **Apple (Liqui-Fruit and Ceres), Secrets of the Valley** (Ceres), **Mango & Orange (Liqui-Fruit), Mysteries of the Mountain (Ceres)**, freshly squeezed grapefruit juice, **Peach and Orange (Liqui-Fruit), Tangerine Teaser (Liqui-Fruit)**. Important: Watch portion sizes as fruit juice is very concentrated!

Trufuco fruit bars (plum, peach, apricot and mixed fruit)

Vegetables

Mediterranean Peppadews (Italyjoe) – calculated

Most vegetables, except for intermediate- and high-GI ones (see Intermediate GI [page 225] and High GI [page 227])

Snacks/Sugars

Litesse Ultra (ultra-refined polydextrose), Litesse II (refined polydextrose), lactitol, xylitol, sorbitol, maltitol and lactose (sugar and/or flour substitutes)

Fructose (should only be consumed in quantities of < 20 g/day, due to the danger of retinal damage);

Sugar-free boiled/jelly sweets, sweetened with fructose, sorbitol, maltitol, lactitol, xylitol or polydextrose

Sugar-free chocolate*

Sugar-free jam, sweetened with fructose, sorbitol, maltitol, lactitol, xylitol or polydextrose

Sponge cake (Australian)

Fine Form fig bar

Apple & Sultana muffins (Muffin Mate) – only available in Cape Town

Fine Form jams, i.e. Apricot, Berry and Seville Orange Marmalade

Strawberry jam (Weigh-Less)

Plain chocolate*/milk chocolate*

Carob (chocolate substitute) – estimated

Cooled low-fat and fat-free custard (sweetened with sugar)

Hot low-fat and fat-free custard (unsweetened/artificially sweetened)

Crisps (packets)*, e.g. Simba, Willards, etc.

Health Rusks (see page 118, *Eating for Sustained Energy,* by Liesbet Delport and Gabi Steenkamp)

Popcorn (homemade, air-popped, i.e. low-fat)

Biscuits (oat)*

Drinks

Sugar-free cooldrink

Biozest Drink

Vitrace MRF (energy drink) Important: Please keep to portions prescribed on packaging, due to its relatively high fructose content)

Sustagen

Dietmax prepared with skimmed/fat-free milk (Biomax product)

Ensure

Ultra Glycem X (calculated in USA)

Miscellaneous

Chutney, average – calculated

Intermediate GI (56 – 69)

Dairy

Mega Lite ice cream (Dairymaid) (11,3 g fat per portion)
Full-cream ice cream*
Condensed milk*

Cereals and porridge (GI lower when eaten with milk)

Mealiemeal, reheated/added corn
Trail Muesli (see page 30, *Eating for Sustained Energy*)
Tropical Fruit Muesli (see page 34, *Eating for Sustained Energy*)
Fruit & Nut Muesli (see page 28, *Eating for Sustained Energy*)
**Oats, raw and cooked (Bokomo/Woolworths/Pick 'n Pay No
  Name Brand)**
Strawberry Pops (Kelloggs)
Fruitful All-bran Flakes (Kelloggs)
Pronutro Flakes, with or without low-fat milk (Bokomo)
Tastee Wheat (semolina)
Chocolate Pronutro (Bokomo) with low-fat milk – calculated
Corn Pops (Kelloggs)
Frosties (Kelloggs)
Choco's (Kelloggs)
All-bran Flakes (Kelloggs)
Shredded Wheat

Bread and flour

Pita bread, i.e. unleavened flat bread
Bran and Oat Bread and Bread rolls (see pages 28-34, *Eating for
  Sustained Energy*)
Rye bread/flour (wheat-free)
Ryvita
Oats (Bokomo/Woolworths/Pick 'n Pay No Name Brand)
Rolled barley
Croissants*
Crumpets*/Griddle cakes* (Australian)

Starches

Sweetcorn (canned)

Basmati and Tasmati rice (white and brown)
Stiff mealiemeal with dried green leaf stew
Baby/new potatoes (with skin)
Couscous
Brown rice
Samp & beans (hot)
Pea soup (homemade and canned)

Fruit

Tropical fruit (fresh), e.g. banana (green bananas have a lower GI), mangoes, pawpaw, papino, guavas (estimated), litchis and pineapple (only have small portions of dried tropical fruits after exercise, as they are very concentrated)

Sultanas, raisins, currants (estimated), dates (estimated), dried fruit cake mix (calculated) and dried fruit flakes (calculated)

Peaches canned in syrup
Apricots canned in syrup
Rock melon (Australian)

Fruit juices: Freshly squeezed orange juice, **Whispers of Summer (Ceres), Apricot (Liqui-Fruit), Orange (Ceres and Liqui-Fruit), Breakfast Punch (Liqui-Fruit), Cranberry & Kiwi (Ceres), Ruby Grapefruit (Ceres), Peach (Ceres), Mango (Ceres), Papaya/Carrot Junior (Ceres), Summer Pine (Liqui-Fruit), Orange (Liqui-Fruit), Berry Blaze (Liqui-Fruit), Cranberry Cooler (Liqui-Fruit), Litchi (Liqui-Fruit), Red Grape (Liqui-Fruit), Hanepoot (Ceres)** Note: Watch portion sizes; juice is very concentrated!

Vegetables

Beetroot
Marog (imifino)/spinach

Snacks/sugars

Pizza with a lower-fat, low-GI topping, e.g. mozzarella cheese, ham and mushrooms
Bran muffins*
Water biscuits (Australian)
Biscuits (shortbread)*
Homewheat Digestive Biscuits

Bran & Raisin Breakfast Bar (Bokomo)

Biscuits (lower fat) containing oat bran/oats/oatmeal, etc. (see pages 118 – 120, *Eating for Sustained Energy*)

Rusks (lower fat) containing oat bran/oats/oatmeal, etc. (see page 120, *Eating for Sustained Energy*)

Muffins/pancakes/crumpets (lower fat) containing low-GI fruit/oats/oat bran, etc. (see pages 30-38, *Eating for Sustained Energy*)

Tart/cake/pudding (lower fat) (see pages 106-116, *Eating for Sustained Energy*)

Pure/raw honey

Jam (average, homemade, minimum of 50% fruit)

Fibre Energy Bar (GNLD)

Standard jelly (based on the GI of sugar)

Sugar/sucrose (table sugar), white and loose brown sugar

Ice lollies (made from sweetened cooldrink)

Instant pudding (dry powder) – calculated

Pear and Raisin Muffin (Muffin Mate) – only available in Cape Town

Bar One/Mars Bar*

Drinks

Nestlé Build Up, vanilla flavour (based on Australian equivalent)

Soft drinks, sweetened with sugar, e.g. Coke, Fanta, cordials, etc.

High GI (70 and above)

Cereals and porridge (GI lower when eaten with milk)

Weetbix (standard and sugar-free) and **Nutrific**

Oats, Instant (plain)

Oat bran, cooked (Jungle)

Oats, raw and cooked (Jungle and Tiger)

Mealiemeal, refined and unrefined (with or without sugar)

Mealiemeal with skimmed milk and sugar

Toasted Muesli Bran (Kelloggs)

Puffed Wheat

Crunchy Nut Cornflakes

Pronutro (Strawberry, Banana, Whole-wheat Honeymelt, Original and Chocolate)
Rice Krispies (Kelloggs)
Honey O's (Kelloggs)
Fermented sorghum porridge
Coco Pops (Kelloggs)
Cornflakes (Kelloggs)
Fruit Loops (Kelloggs)
Mabella porridge (with and without sugar)
Special K (Kelloggs)
Oats, Instant (flavoured) – very high GI

Starches

White rice, especially "sticky" rice
Millet
Normal-sized potatoes (with or without skins) – baked, fried, microwaved, mashed, instant (i.e. Smash), oven chips and French fries*/slap chips*/hot chips*
All pasta made from wheat, potato or rice flour, as well as 2-Minute Noodles
Samp and mealie rice
Mealiemeal, unrefined and refined, including polenta
Stiff mealiemeal and nkaka (dried green leaf stew)

Bread and flour

All brown, white and standard wholewheat bread (those containing few, or no, kernels), Nutty Wheat bread, as well as all bread rolls, bagels, hot cross buns, Melba toast, gluten-free bread, etc.
Most flours, i.e. cornflour, cake flour, bread flour, as well as whole-wheat flour (Nutty Wheat), potato flour, rice flour, etc., as well as soup powder (high in sodium) and gravy powder – estimated
Plain scones and muffins
Cream Crackers – estimated
Rice Cakes (white and brown)
Snackbread (refined and wholewheat), Crackerbread, etc.

Fruit

All melons, including sweet melon and watermelon
Fruit juices: **Medley of Fruit (Ceres) and Litchi (Ceres)**

Vegetables

Green beans with potato
Turnips
Parsnips
Carrots and carrot juice
Pumpkin, Hubbard squash, butternut (yellow or winter pump-
    kins/squash) (Australian)

Snacks/sugars

Sweets (boiled, jelly type, marshmallows, toffees, etc.)
Corn chips* (similar to SA Fritos)
Cream Crackers – estimated
Energy Bars, Strawberry (PVM)
Swiss roll, jam
Tapioca made with milk
Wafer biscuits
Marie Biscuits
Boudoir Biscuits – calculated
Commercial honey and syrup
Glucose and dextrose
Maltose and maltodextrin
Sugar-free jelly with maltodextrin as main ingredient – very
    high GI!
Tofu (frozen dairy-free dessert)

Drinks

Energy/sports drinks, e.g. Game, Energade, Powerade, Lucozade
    and Lucozade Sport

Alphabetical Glycemic Index Ratings of some South African foods

Key

bold   These products have been tested in South Africa by
              GIFSA

*   High fat foods. These products do not comply with
              GIFSA's and the Heart Foundation of South Africa's
              standard's for a lower-fat product.

Calculated   Theoretical calculation done by Liesbet Delport (ED)
              and Gabi Steenkamp (GS)

Estimated   Estimated values based on extensive experience in GI
              testing and developing low-GI, lower-fat recipes (by ED
              and GS).

A	GI RATING
All-bran Flakes with skimmed milk	Low
All-bran Flakes, Kelloggs (no milk)	Intermediate
Apple & Cinnamon Low-GI Muesli, Nature's Source	Low
Apple Juice, LiquiFruit and Ceres	Low
Apple, canned (estimated)	Low
Apple, dried (estimated)	Intermediate
Apple, fresh	Low
Apricot jam, Fine Form and homemade	Low
Apricot Juice, LiquiFruit	Intermediate
Apricot, canned in apricot juice (estimated)	Low
Apricots, canned in syrup	Intermediate
Apricot, dried	Low
Apricots, raw	Low

B	
Baby/new potato, with skin	Intermediate
Bagels	**High**
Baked beans, in tomato sauce	Low
Banana, green	Low
Banana, ripe	Intermediate
Bar One/Mars Bar* **(high fat)**	Intermediate
Barley, pearled, boiled or cracked	Low
Basmati rice	Intermediate
Beans and samp	Intermediate
Beans, (dried) stew	Low
Beans, baked beans in tomato sauce	Low
Beans, barlotti	Low
Beans, black-eyed	Low
Beans, black-eyed peas	Low
Beans, brown	Low
Beans, butter	Low
Beans, cannellini	Low
Beans, chickpeas, cooked or canned	Low
Beans, green with potato	**High**
Beans, green, fresh or canned	Low
Beans, haricot	Low
Beans, kidney, cooked or canned	Low
Beans, lentils	Low

230

Beans, mixed, average	Low
Beans, red	Low
Beans, small white	Low
Beans, soya, cooked or canned	Low
Beans, split peas	Low
Beans, sugar	Low
Beetroot	Intermediate
Biozest cooldrink	Low
Biscuit, Boudoir (calculated)	**High**
Biscuit, Bran Crisp Bread	Low
Biscuit, Cream Cracker * (estimated)	**High**
Biscuit, Digestive Homewheat	Intermediate
Biscuit, Marie	**High**
Biscuit, Provita, multigrain and original	Low
Biscuit, Ryevita	Low
Bisto, gravy powder	**High**
Bokomo Maximize, Cereal	Low
Bokomo Morning Harvest Muesli	Low
Bokomo Oats, cooked or raw	Intermediate
Bran, Oat bran, Jungle, raw	Low
Bran, Shredded, cereal, Pick 'n Pay	Low
Bread, brown (Standard SA loaf)	**High**
Bread, seedloaf bread, Uncle Salie's Homemade and others	Low
Bread, pita, i.e. unleavened flat bread	Intermediate
Bread, rye, wheat-free	Intermediate
Bread, white (Standard SA loaf / high fibre)	**High**
Bread, wholewheat, (standard SA loaf)	**High**
Bread roll	**High**
Brown beans (sugar beans)	Low
Brown bread (SA standard loaf)	**High**
Brown bread, sliced, Fine Form	Low
Brown rice	Intermediate
Brown rice with lentils	Low
Brown Seedloaf bread, Uncle's Salie's Homemade and others	Low
Brown sugar, loose	Intermediate
Buckwheat	Low

Build-up, Nestlé, vanilla (estimated from Australian value)	Intermediate
Butterbeans	Low
Buttermilk* (usually full cream in South Africa, check label)	Low

C

Cake flour	**High**
Cake mix (mixed dried fruit for baking)	Intermediate
Cake, Swiss roll (jam)	**High**
Carbonated drinks (e.g. Fanta, Coke)	Intermediate
Carob, chocolate substitute (calculated)	Low
Carrots	Intermediate – **High**
Cereals (**note:** the GI will be lowered when eaten with milk)	
Cereal, Bokomo Maximize	Low
Cereal, Bokomo Morning Harvest Muesli	Low
Cereal, Fine Form Muesli	Low
Cereal, Kelloggs All-bran Flakes	Intermediate
Cereal, Kelloggs All-bran with skim milk	Low
Cereal, Kelloggs Choco's	Intermediate
Cereal, Kelloggs Coco Pops	**High**
Cereal, Kelloggs Corn Pops	Intermediate
Cereal, Kelloggs Cornflakes	**High**
Cereal, Kelloggs Crunchy Nut Cornflakes	**High**
Cereal, Kelloggs Frosties	Intermediate
Cereal, Kelloggs Fruit loops	**High**
Cereal, Kelloggs Fruitful All-Bran Flakes	Intermediate
Cereal, Kelloggs Hi-Fibre Bran	Low
Cereal, Kelloggs Honey O's	**High**
Cereal, Kelloggs Nutrific	**High**
Cereal, Kelloggs Rice Krispies	**High**
Cereal, Kelloggs Special K	**High**
Cereal, Kelloggs Strawberry Pops	Intermediate
Cereal, Kelloggs Toasted Muesli Bran	**High**
Cereal, Maximize, Bokomo	Low
Cereal, Nature's Source Apple and Cinnamon muesli	Low
Cereal, Nature's Source Mixed Berry Muesli	Low

Cereal, Nature's Source Orange and Mixed Spices Muesli	Low
Cereal, Pick 'n Pay Shredded Bran	Low
Cereal, Pronutro Chocolate	High
Cereal, Pronutro Chocolate with low-fat milk (calculated)	Intermediate
Cereal, Pronutro Flakes	Intermediate
Cereal, Pronutro Flakes with low-fat milk	Intermediate
Cereal, Pronutro Original	High
Cereal, Pronutro Original with low-fat milk	Low
Cereal, Pronutro Strawberry	High
Cereal, Pronutro, Whole-wheat, Apple bake	Low
Cereal, Pronutro, Whole-wheat, Honeymelt	High
Cereal, Pronutro, Whole-wheat, Original	Low
Cereal, Pronutro, Whole-wheat with low-fat milk	Low
Cereal, Puffed wheat	High
Cereal, Shredded Bran, Pick 'n Pay	Low
Cereal, Shredded wheat	Intermediate
Cereal, Weetbix	High
Cereal, Weetbix, sugar-free	High
Ceres, Apple Juice	Low
Ceres, Berry Blaze Juice	Intermediate
Ceres, Cranberry and Kiwi Juice	Intermediate
Ceres, Hanepoot Grape Juice	Intermediate
Ceres, Litchi Juice	High
Ceres, Mango Juice	Intermediate
Ceres, Medley of Fruits Juice	High
Ceres, Mysteries of the Mountain Juice	Low
Ceres, Orange Juice	Intermediate
Ceres, Peach Juice	Intermediate
Ceres, Rubi Grapefruit Juice	Intermediate
Ceres, Secrets of the Valley Juice	Low
Ceres, Whispers of Summer Juice	Intermediate
Cheese pizza	Intermediate
Cherries, fresh	Low
Chick peas, dried or canned	Low
Chips, hot* **(high fat)**	High
Chips/crisps* (corn), similar to SA Fritos **(high fat)**	High
Chips/crisps* (eg, Simba, Willards) **(high fat)**	Low

Chocolate, milk* slab **(high fat)**	Low
Chocolate, plain* slab **(high fat)**	Low
Chocolate, sugar-free* slab **(high fat)**	Low
Chocolate Ice cream (Fine Form) (5g fat/100g)	Low
Chocolate Pronutro	**High**
Choco's, Kelloggs	Intermediate
Chutney, average (calculated)	Low
Coco Pops, Kelloggs	
Coke, carbonated beverage	Intermediate
Commercial honey	**High**
Condensed milk	Intermediate
Cooldrink cordial (e.g. Oros)	Intermediate
Corn Thins	**High**
Corn, canned or frozen	Low
Corn crisps (e.g. Fritos)	**High**
Cornflakes, Kelloggs	**High**
Cornflour, Maizena (estimated)	**High**
Corn pops, Kelloggs	Intermediate
Couscous, durum wheat	Intermediate
Cracker, Bran Crisp Bread	Low
Cracker, Cream Cracker* (calculated)	**High**
Crackers, Provita, multigrain and original	Low
Croissants* **(high fat)**	Intermediate
Crumpets* **(high fat)**	Intermediate
Currants	Intermediate
Custard (made from 30 ml custard powder, 30 ml sugar and 500 ml low-fat milk) (calculated) – preferably cooled down	Low

D

Dairymaid Mega Lite Ice cream (11,3g fat per ice cream)	Low
Dates, dried (estimated)	Intermediate
Dextrose/ Polydextrose	Low
Dialite Ice cream	Low
Dietmax, made with skimmed milk	Low
Digestive biscuit	Intermediate
Doughnut* **(high fat)**	**High**
Dried fruit: see under individual fruits	
Durum wheat pasta (average)	Low

E

Energade	**High**
Energy drinks (e.g. Powerade, Energade, Lucozade, Game, Lucozade Sport)	**High**
Ensure	Low

F

Fanta, carbonated beverage	Intermediate
Fat-free flavoured yoghurt	Low
Fibre Bar, GNLD (Golden Products)	Intermediate
Fig bar, Fine Form	Low
Fine Form products	Low
Flavoured milks, low-fat, sweetened and sugar-free	Low
Flour, cake and bread	**High**
Flour, cornflour	**High**
Flour, Nuttywheat/wholewheat cake flour	**High**
Flour, rice	**High**
Flour, rye	Intermediate
Flour, soya (calculated)	Low
Flour, wheat, cake/bread/wholewheat	**High**
FOS (Fructo-oligo-saccharide)	Low
French Fries* **(high fat)**	**High**
Frozen peas	Low
Fructose	Low
Fruitful All-bran Flakes, Kelloggs	Intermediate
Fruit bars, Trufuco (Plum, Peach, Apricot and Mixed Fruit)	Low
Fruit juice, Ceres (Apple, Secrets of the Valley, Mysteries of the Mountain)	Low
Fruit juice, Ceres (Berry Blaze, Cranberry & Kiwi, Mango, Hanepoot, Orange, Peach, Ruby Grapefruit, Whispers of Summer)	Intermediate
Fruit juice, Ceres (Litchi, Medley of Fruits)	**High**
Fruit juice, grapefruit, freshly squeezed	Low
Fruit juice, LiquiFruit (Apple, Mango & Orange, Peach & Orange, Passion Power, Tangerine Teaser)	Low
Fruit juice, LiquiFruit (Apricot, Breakfast Punch, Cranberry Cooler, Litchi, Orange, Red Grape, Summerpine, Passion Power)	Intermediate

Fruit juice, orange, freshly squeezed (average)	Intermediate
Fruit Loops, Kelloggs	**High**
Fruit salad, canned (Canadian)	Low
Fruit salad, dried (calculated)	Intermediate
Fruit salad, fresh (mainly deciduous/citrus fruits)	Low
Fruit, apple, canned (estimated)	Low
Fruit, apple, dried	Intermediate
Fruit, apple, fresh	Low
Fruit, apricot, canned in fruit juice (estimated)	Low
Fruit, apricot, canned in syrup	Intermediate
Fruit, apricot, dried	Low
Fruit, apricot, fresh	Low
Fruit, banana, fresh, green	Low
Fruit, banana, fresh, ripe	Intermediate
Fruit, cherries, fresh	Low
Fruit, dates, dried (estimated)	Intermediate
Fruit, dried cake mix (calculated)	Intermediate
Fruit, grapefruit	Low
Fruit, grapes	Low
Fruit, kiwifruit	Low
Fruit, mango	Intermediate
Fruit, orange	Low
Fruit, papino	Intermediate
Fruit, paw-paw	Intermediate
Fruit, peach, fresh	Low
Fruit, pear, fresh or canned in fruit juice	Low
Fruit, pineapple, fresh or canned in fruit juice/syrup	Intermediate
Fruit, plum, fresh	Low
Fruit, raisins, dried	Intermediate
Fruit, strawberries	Low
Fruit, sultana, dried	Intermediate
Fruit, watermelon, fresh	**High**

G

Game, sportsdrink	**High**
Glucose	**High**
GNLD, Fibre energy bar	Intermediate
Grapefruit, fresh	Low

Grapefruit, juice, freshly squeezed	Low
Grape juice (LiquiFruit, Ceres)	Intermediate
Grapes, fresh	Low
Gravy powder (e.g. Bisto, Gravo), (calculated)	**High**
Green beans	Low
Green mealies	Low
Green peas	Low

H

Haricot beans	Low
Health bars, GNLD Fibre Energy Bar	Intermediate
Health bars, PVM, Strawberry bar	High
Health bars, PVM, Zone bar	Low
Hi-Fibre Bran, Kelloggs	Low
Homewheat Digestive Biscuits	Intermediate
Honey O's, Kelloggs	High
Honey, commercial	**High**
Honey, raw	Intermediate
Hot cross buns	**High**

I

Ice cream, chocolate (5g fat/100g), Fine Form	Low
Ice cream, Dairymaid Mega Lite (11,3g fat per ice cream)	Low
Ice cream, Dialite (fat-free)	Low
Ice cream*, full-cream **(high fat)**	Intermediate
Ice cream, low-fat (average)	Low
Instant noodles (South African)	**High**
Instant oats, flavoured	VERY High
Instant oats, natural	High
Instant potato (e.g. Smash)	**High**
Instant pudding, dry powder (calculated)	Intermediate

J

Jam, Apricot (Fine Form)	Low
Jam, average, homemade (at least 50% fruit)	Intermediate
Jam, Marmalade, Seville Orange (Fine Form)	Low
Jam, Strawberry (Weighless)	Low
Jelly (based on GI of sugar)	Intermediate

Jelly, sugar-free, with maltodextrin as main ingredient	**VERY high**
Juice, see fruit juice	
Jungle Oat Bran, raw	Low
Jungle Oats, raw or cooked	**High**

K

Kelloggs All-bran Flakes	Intermediate
Kelloggs All-bran with skim milk	Low
Kelloggs Choco's	Intermediate
Kelloggs Coco Pops	**High**
Kelloggs Corn Pops	Intermediate
Kelloggs Cornflakes	**High**
Kelloggs Crunchy Nut Cornflakes	**High**
Kelloggs Frosties	Intermediate
Kelloggs Fruit Loops	**High**
Kelloggs Fruitful All-Bran Flakes	Intermediate
Kelloggs Hi-Fibre Bran	Low
Kelloggs Honey O's	**High**
Kelloggs Nutrific	**High**
Kelloggs Rice Krispies	**High**
Kelloggs Special K	**High**
Kelloggs Strawberry Pops	Intermediate
Kelloggs Toasted Muesli Bran	**High**
Kidney beans, including large, white and canned	Low
Kiwifruit, fresh	Low

L

Lactitol (sugar substitute)	Low
Lactose (milk sugar)	Low
Lasagne, Fine Form	Low
Legumes, all dry beans, peas and lentils	Low
Legumes, baked beans	Low
Lentil soup, canned	Low
Lentils	Low
LiquiFruit Apple Juice	Low
LiquiFruit Apricot Juice	Intermediate
LiquiFruit Berry Blaze	Intermediate
LiquiFruit Breakfast Punch Juice	Intermediate

LiquiFruit Cranberry Cooler Juice	Intermediate
LiquiFruit Litchi Juice	Intermediate
LiquiFruit Mango and Orange Juice	Low
LiquiFruit Orange Juice	Intermediate
LiquiFruit Passion Power Juice	Low
LiquiFruit Peach & Orange Juice	Low
LiquiFruit Red Grape Juice	Intermediate
LiquiFruit Summer Pine Juice	Intermediate
LiquiFruit Tangerine Teaser Juice	Low
Litchi Juice Ceres	**High**
Litchi Juice LiquiFruit	Intermediate
Low-fat ice cream (e.g. Fine Form)	Low
Low-fat milk (2%)	Low
Low-fat yoghurt, plain or fruit flavoured	Low
Lucozade Sport (Sport/Energy drink)	**VERY High**
Luzozade (Sport/Energy drink)	**High**

M

Mabella porridge, with sugar	**High**
Mabella porridge, without sugar	**High**
Macaroni, (Mr Pasta/Pasta Grande)	Low
Maizena (cornflour)	**High**
Maltose	**High**
Mango, fresh	Intermediate
Mango & Orange Juice, LiquiFruit	Low
Mango Juice, Ceres	Intermediate
Marie Biscuit	**High**
Marmalade, Seville Orange, Fine Form	Low
Marog	Intermediate
Mars Bar* / Bar One* **(high fat)**	Intermediate
Marshmallows	**High**
Mashed potato	**High**
Maximize cereal, Bokomo	Low
Mealiemeal, cold	Low
Mealiemeal, sifted (including polenta)	**High**
Mealiemeal, unsifted (including polenta)	**High**
Mealiemeal porridge, cooled down	Low
Mealiemeal porridge, soft, with or without sugar	**High**

Mealiemeal with skim milk and sugar	High
Mealies, green	Low
Medley of Fruits Juice, Ceres	High
Mega Lite Dairymaid Ice cream (11,3g fat per ice cream)	Low
Melba toast	High
Microwaved potatoes	High
Milk, full-cream* (3,5% fat)	Low
Milk, buttermilk (usually full-cream in South Africa)	Low
Milk, flavoured, low-fat (2% fat), sweetened or sugar-free	Low
Milk, low-fat (2% fat)	Low
Milk, skim (0,5% fat)	Low
Milk chocolate* slab **(high fat)**	Low
Millet	High
Minute Noodles	High
Mixed beans, average	Low
Mixed Berry Muesli, Nature's Source	Low
Muesli, Bokomo, Morning Harvest	Low
Muesli, Fine Form	Low
Muesli, Kelloggs, Toasted Muesli Bran	High
Muesli, Nature's Source, Apple and Cinnamon Muesli	Low
Muesli, Nature's Source, Mixed Berry Muesli	Low
Muesli, Nature's Source, Orange and Spices Muesli	Low
Muffin, bran/health* (high fat)	Intermediate

N

Nature's Source, Apple and Cinnamon Muesli	Low
Nature's Source, Mixed Berry Muesli	Low
Nature's Source, Orange and Spices Muesli	Low
New/baby potatoes (with skin)	Intermediate
Noodles, 2-minute (South African)	High
Noodles, instant (South African)	High
Noodles, instant (South African), Durum wheat (estimated)	Intermediate
Nutrific, Kelloggs	High
Nutty wheat flour (estimated)	High

O

Oat bran, cooked (Jungle)	High

Oat bran, raw (Jungle)	Low
Oats, Bokomo, raw or cooked	Intermediate
Oats, Instant, Oats-so-easy, flavours	VERY High
Oats, Instant, Oats-so-easy, natural	High
Oats, Jungle, raw or cooked	High
Oats, Pick 'n Pay, raw or cooked	Intermediate
Oats, Tiger, raw or cooked	High
Oats, Woolworths, raw or cooked	Intermediate
Oats-so-easy, flavours	VERY High
Oats-so-easy, natural	High
Orange and Spice Muesli, Nature's Source	Low
Orange, fresh	Low
Orange juice, average, freshly squeezed	Intermediate
Orange Juice, Ceres & LiquiFruit	Intermediate
Original Pronutro	High
Original Pronutro with low-fat milk	Low
Oros, cordial	Intermediate

P

Papaya/Carrot Junior Juice (Ceres)	Intermediate
Papino/Papaya, fresh	Intermediate
Parsnips	High
Pasta, homemade with flour	High
Pasta, lasagne, Fine Form	Low
Pasta, macaroni (Mr Pasta/Pasta Grande)	Low
Pasta, spaghetti (Mr Pasta/Pasta Grande)	Low
Pasta, tagliatelle (plain, wholewheat & spinach), Fine Form	Low
Paw-paw, fresh	Intermediate
Pea soup, canned	Intermediate
Pea soup, homemade	Intermediate
Peach, fresh or canned in fruit juice	Low
Peach, canned in syrup	Intermediate
Pear, fresh or canned in fruit juice	Low
Pearled barley	Low
Pearled wheat (stampkoring)	Low
Peas, chickpeas, canned and dry cooked	Low
Peas, dried or black-eyed	Low

Peas, green, fresh or frozen	Low
Peas, snap (mangetout)	Low
Peas, split	Low
Peppadews, Mediterranean, Italyjoe (calculated)	Low
Pick 'n Pay, Oats, raw or cooked	Intermediate
Pick 'n Pay, shredded bran cereal	Low
Pineapple, fresh or canned in pineapple juice/syrup	Intermediate
Pita bread, i.e. unleavened flat bread	Intermediate
Pizza, cheese	Intermediate
Plain chocolate* slab **(high fat)**	Low
Plain yoghurt, low-fat	Low
Plums, fresh	Low
Polenta	**High**
Polydextrose	Low
Popcorn (low-fat)	Low
Porridge, Mabella, with or without sugar	**High**
Porridge, mealiemeal, sifted and unsifted	**High**
Porridge, mealiemeal, cold	Low
Porridge, Oatbran, cooked	**High**
Porridge, Oatbran, raw	Low
Porridge, Oats, Bokomo, cooked	Intermediate
Porridge, Oats, Jungle, raw or cooked	**High**
Porridge, Oats, Pick 'n Pay, raw or cooked	Intermediate
Porridge, Oats, Tiger, raw or cooked	**High**
Porridge, Oats, Woolworths, cooked	Intermediate
Porridge, Oat-so-easy, flavours	**VERY High**
Porridge, Oat-so-easy, natural	**High**
Porridge, Pronutro (see under Pronutro below)	
Porridge, soft mealiemeal, with or without sugar	**High**
Porridge, soft mealiemeal with skim milk and sugar	**High**
Potatoes and green beans	**High**
Potatoes, baby/new (with skin)	Intermediate
Potatoes, baked	**High**
Potatoes, chips, hot* **(high fat)**	**High**
Potatoes, instant (e.g. Smash)	**High**
Potatoes, mashed	**High**
Potatoes, microwaved	**High**
Potatoes, new (with skin)	Intermediate

Potatoes, roasted without fat	**High**
Potatoes, sweet (Australian)	Low
Powerade, sportsdrink	**High**
Pronutro, Chocolate	**High**
Pronutro, Chocolate with milk (calculated)	Intermediate
Pronutro, Flakes	Intermediate
Pronutro, Flakes with low-fat milk	Intermediate
Pronutro, Original	**High**
Pronutro, Original with low-fat milk	Low
Pronutro, Strawberry	**High**
Pronutro, Whole-wheat, Apple bake	Low
Pronutro, Whole-wheat, Honeymelt	**High**
Pronutro, Whole-wheat, Original	Low
Provita, multigrain and original	Low
Prunes, dried	Low
Pudding, instant powder (calculated)	Intermediate
Pudding, jelly (based on GI of sugar)	Intermediate
Pudding, sugar-free jelly, with maltodextrin as main ingredient	**VERY high**
Puffed wheat	**High**
Pumpernickel, wholegrain rye bread	Low
Pumpkins (Australian)	**High**
PVM, Strawberry bar	**High**
PVM, Zone bar	Low

R

Raisins	Intermediate
Red beans	Low
Red Grape Juice, LiquiFruit	Intermediate
Rice, basmati	Intermediate
Rice, bran (25% fibre, 20% oil)	Low
Rice, brown	Intermediate – **High**
Rice, brown with lentils	Low
Rice, Tastic	Low
Rice, wheat (pearled wheat)	Low
Rice, wild	Intermediate – Low

Rice, especially "sticky" rice (estimated)	**High**
Rice cakes	**High**
Rice flour	**High**
Rice Krispies, Kelloggs	**High**
Roast potatoes *(high fat)	**High**
Rolled barley	Intermediate
Ruby Grapefruit Juice, Ceres	Intermediate
Rusks, commercial	**High**
Rye bread	Intermediate
Rye flour	Intermediate
Ryvita	Intermediate

S

Samp	**High**
Samp and beans	Intermediate
Samp, cold	Low
Seedloaf bread, Uncle Salie's Homemade breads	Low
Shredded bran cereal, Pick 'n Pay	Low
Skim milk	Low
Slap chips (French fries)* **(high fat)**	**High**
Small white beans	Low
Smash, instant mashed potato	**High**
Snackbread, wholewheat	**High**
Snap peas (mangetout)	Low
Soft drinks (e.g. Coke, Fanta)	Intermediate
Soup powder and instant soups (estimated)	**High**
Soya beans	Low
Soya flour (calculated)	Low
Spaghetti (durum wheat)	Low
Special K, Kelloggs	**High**
Spinach	Intermediate
Split peas	Low
Sports drinks (e.g. Energade, Game, Powerade)	**High**
Sports drink, Vitrace (MRF); not suitable for after exercise	Low
Stampkoring (pearled wheat)	Low
Strawberries	Low
Strawberry jam (Weighless)	Low

Sucrose	Intermediate
Sugar beans	Low
Sugar, white	Intermediate
Sugar-free chocolate *(high fat)	Low
Sugar-free jelly, with maltodextrin as main ingredient	**VERY High**
Sugar-free fat-free yoghurt (Clover Danone)	Low
Sugar-free Weetbix	**High**
Sugar, brown, loose	Intermediate
Sultanas	Intermediate
Sustagen, Meal-in-a-glass	Low
Sweetcorn, whole, fresh, canned or frozen	Low
Sweet potato (Australian)	Low
Swiss roll, jam	**High**

T

Table sugar	Intermediate
Tagliatelle (plain, wholewheat & spinach), Fine Form	Low
Tapioca, with milk	**High**
Tastic rice	Low
Tiger, Oats, raw or cooked	**High**
Toast, brown, wholewheat or white bread	**High**
Tomato soup made with milk (not cream)	Low
Turnips	**High**
Two-minute noodles (South African)	**High**

U

Ultra GlycemX (calculated in USA)	Low
Uncle Salie's Homemade Brown Seedloaf	Low

V

Vegetables, see individual vegetables in list	Mostly low
Vitrace, Energy drink (MRF); not suitable for after exercise	Low

W

Waffles	**High**
Watermelon, fresh	**High**
Weetbix, Bokomo	**High**

Weetbix, sugar-free, Bokomo	**High**
Wheat flour (cake flour)	**High**
Wheat rice (pearled wheat)	Low
White beans, cooked	Low
White bread (standard SA loaf)	**High**
White rice, estimated (especially "sticky" rice)	**High**
White sugar	Intermediate
Wholewheat bread	**High**
Whole-wheat Pronutro, Honeymelt	**High**
Whole-wheat Pronutro, Original and Apple Bake	Low
Wholewheat snackbread	**High**
Wild rice	Intermediate – Low
Woolworths, Oats, raw or cooked	Intermediate

X

Xylitol (sugar substitute)	Low

Y

Yoghurt, (fat-free fruit, all flavours), Clover Danone	Low
Yoghurt, low-fat, fruit	Low
Yoghurt, low-fat, sugar-free	Low
Yoghurt, plain, low-fat	Low

References

Brand Miller, J. et al. (1996) *The GI Factor. The Glycemic Index Solution.* Hodder and Stoughton, Australia.

Cullen, K.W., Dr PH, RD; Baranowski, T., Phd; Smith, S.P., RD (2001) "Using goal setting as a strategy for dietary behaviour change" in *Journal of the American Dietetic Association,* 101 (5): 562-566.

Delport, L. en Steenkamp, G. (2000) *Eating for Sustained Energy.* Tafelberg Publishers, Cape Town.

De Marco, H.M., Sucher, K.P., Cisar, C.J. and Butterfield, G.E. (1999) "Pre-exercise carbohydrate meals: effects of glycemic index" in *Medicine and Science in Sports and Exercise,* 31 (1): 164-170.

Garg, A. (1998) "High monosaturated fat diets for patients with diabetes: a meta-analysis" in *American Journal of Clinical Nutrition,* 67 (supplement): 5 775-5 825.

Green, M., Wales, J.K., Lawton, C.L. en Blundell, J.E. (2000) "Comparison of high-fat and high-carbohydrate foods in a meal or snack in short-term fat and energy intakes in obese women" in *British Journal of Nutrition,* 84 (4): 521-553.

Hampton, D. (1984) *The diet alternative.* Whitaker House, USA.

Jeukendrup, A.E., Thielen, J.J.H.C., Wagenmakers, A.J.M. et al. (1998) "Sports nutrition" in *American Journal of Clinical Nutrition,* 67: 397-404.

Katan, M., Grundy, S. and Willet, W. (1997) "Beyond low-fat diets" in *New England Journal of Medicine,* 337: 563-566.

Kirk, T.R., Burkill, S. and Cursitor, M.C. (1997) "Dietary fat reduction achieved by increasing consumption of starchy food – an intervention study" in *European Journal of Clinical Nutrition,* 51: 455-461.

Life, J.D.R. (2001) "Performance nutrition" in *Muscle Media,* July/August, Chapt. 18, p.18.8.

Meyer, V.J. et al. (1988) *Die fisiologiese basis van geneeskunde.* Fourth revised edition. HAUM, Pretoria.

Pollock, M.L., Wilmore, J.H. and Fox, S.M. (1978) *Health and Fitness through Physical Activity.* John Wiley & Sons.

Prentice, A.M. (1997) "Obesity: the inevitable penalty of civilization?" in *British Medical Bulletin,* 53: 229-237.

Raben, A. (2001) *Sucrose vs Starch: Different Effects on Body Weight, Lipidemia and Glycemia.* GI Workshop.

Rosal, M.C., Ebbeling, C.B., Ockdene, I.S. and Hebert, J.R. (2001) "Facilitating Dietary Change: The Patient-centered Counseling Model" in *Journal of the American Dietetic Association,* 101(3): 332-341.

Saris, W.H.M. (1998) "Fit, fat and fat free: the metabolic aspects of weight control" in *International Journal for Obesity,* 22 (supplement): 515-521.

Sparks, M.J., Selig, S.S. and Febraraio, M.A. (1998) "Glycemic index and endurance performance" in *Medicine and Science in Sports and Exercise,* 30 (6): 844–849.

Steenkamp, G. and Delport, L. (2002) *The South African Glycemic Index Guide.* Glycemic Index Foundation of South Africa.

Stoppard, M. (ed.) (1980) *The Face and Body Book.* Frances Lincoln Publishers, London, p. 151-161.

Utter, A.C. et al. (1999) "Carbohydrate intake and perceived exertion during exercise" in *European Journal of Applied Physiology,* 80: 92-99.

Wee, S.L., Williams, C., Gray, S. and Horabin, J. (1999) "High and low glycemic index and endurance running capacity" in *Medicine and Science in Sports and Exercise,* 31: 393-399.

WHO. (1998) "Obesity: preventing and managing the global epidemic" in WHO/NUT/NCD/98.1.

General index

Index of recipes

see also Meals for a week 157–166